To My Friend

WM. J. HERRMANN

who knows more about all kinds of manly sports
and health-giving exercise than any other living
man.

1

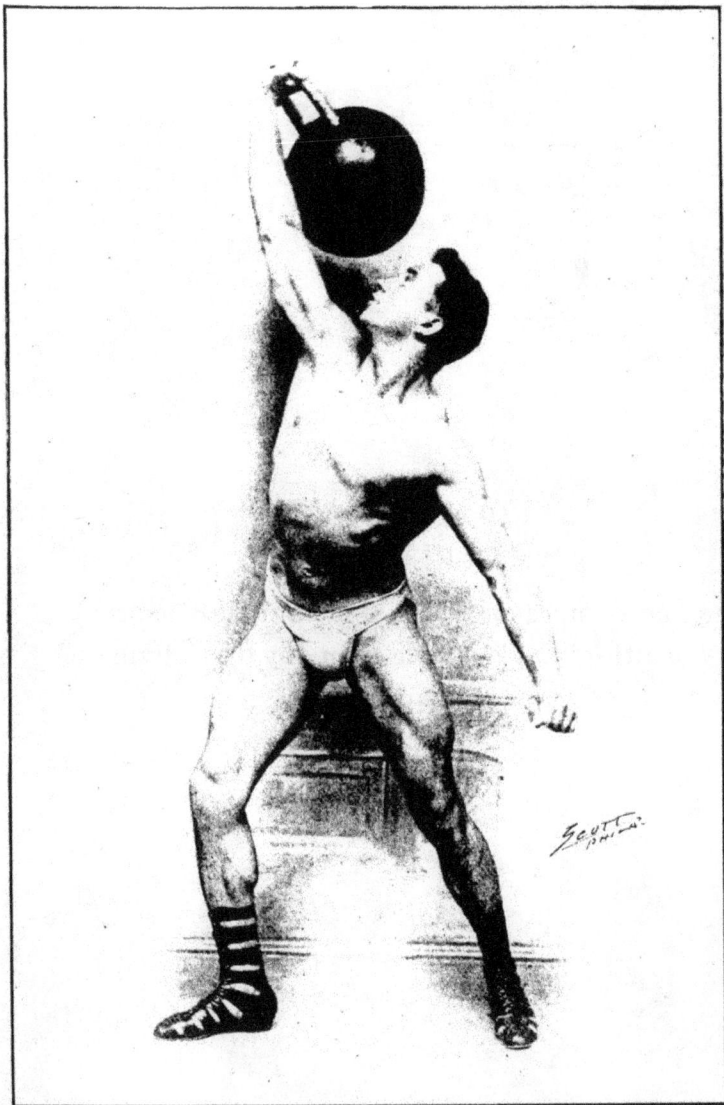

Fig. 65

Frontispiece, Figure 65, Anton Matysek finishing a "One-Arm Swing" with a kettle-bell.

SUPERSTRENGTH

By

ALAN CALVERT

Former Editor of the Strength Magazine

Originally Published in 1924

PUBLISHED BY O'Faolain Patriot LLC, Copyright 2012

info@PhysicalCultureBooks.com

Published in the United States of America

ISBN-13: 978-1475153224

ISBN-10: 1475153228

To Order More Copies Visit: Physical Culture Books.com

TABLE OF CONTENTS

CHAPTER I

INTRODUCTORY

One day, several years ago, I took a professional "Strong Man" named Herold into my factory to inquire about a special bar-bell which he had ordered. In order to make the particular kind of bell he wanted, we had to fit a piece of hollow pipe over a solid steel bar. Just before we entered the shop, one of the workmen had started to drive the bar through the piece of pipe; but there must have been some obstruction inside the pipe, because the bar stuck half-way. The workman was about to put the pipe in a vise so that he could remove the bar, when "Herold" intervened. He grasped one end of the pipe in his right hand, and told the workman to take hold of the projecting steel bar and pull it out. The "Strong Man" stood with his right foot slightly advanced, and his right elbow close to his side. The workman, who was a husky fellow, took hold of the projecting steel rod in both his hands and gave several tremendous heaves; but although he used every part of his weight and strength, he could not pull the bar out of the pipe. So I added my weight to his, and by a great effort we managed to draw the bar out. Meanwhile "Herold" stood as though he were carved out of bronze. Even when both of us were pulling against him we never shook him a particle, and neither did we draw his right elbow a fraction of an inch from his side. He held the end of the iron pipe in his hand just as securely as though it had been put in the vise. I want you to bear this story in mind, for I will refer to it several times later on in this book. At this time, I wish to use it as an illustration of the difference between arm strength, and general bodily strength.

When the author of a novel wishes to give his readers an idea of the hero's strength, he says that his hero is "as strong as two or three ordinary men." That is one of those statements which is very easy to make and very hard to prove. In the first place, it raises in your mind the question, "How strong is the ordinary man?" That is something that no one can tell you. In order to know the answer, it would be necessary to test at least 100,000 men at exactly the same stunts and under exactly the same conditions. All I can tell you is that the average man is not half as strong as he ought to be, or as he could be if he were properly trained.

Now, take the case of the "Strong Man" referred to above. Undoubtedly that man could out-pull any two ordinary men, although he weighed but 160 lbs., and the two of us, who pulled against him, weighed 175 lbs. apiece. If you, who read this book, had seen this "Strong Man," you would have at once exclaimed about his marvellous arms, which measured nearly 17 inches around the biceps; and it is equally probable that you would have ascribed all his strength to his arms. But his right arm, mighty as it was, was doing only part of the work in pulling against us. It was the great strength of the muscles on the right side of his upper back which enabled him to keep his right elbow against his side. If he had been weak in the back, we would have toppled him over on his face at the first pull; but his back was so strong that we could not make him bend forward the least trifle at the waist. If his legs had been weak, we would have slid him along the floor, while as a matter of fact, his feet gripped the ground so strongly that we could not budge him an inch from his original position.

Now, this man was stronger than two average men. In fact, he was probably about as strong as two lumbermen weighing 200 lbs. each. (I had many opportunities to observe his prodigious power.) In a private gymnasium in Buffalo, there was a strength- testing device in the form of an old-fashioned wagon spring. This spring was placed a few inches above the floor in its normal position; a chain with a handle was fastened to the lower arm of the spring; and the athlete whose strength was to be tested straddled the spring and pulled upward on the chain, so as to bring the two sides of the spring closer together. Across the middle of the spring was a gauge graduated in one-sixteenths of an inch. This test gave a good idea of the ability of a man to raise heavy weights from the ground. The ordinary man could compress the spring about three-eighths of an inch. Some very strong workmen had compressed it to as much as three-quarters of an inch. Herold compressed it one and one-half inches; and I know that to be a fact, because another "Strong Man" told me that he, himself, had been able to compress it only one and one-quarter inches, and referred to his pull as a record. Now, this first lifter (Herold) was not by any means the strongest man in the world; although he was one of the very best in his class. He weighed about 160 lbs., and was just about as strong as either Herman or Kurt Saxon; and while most of his lifting records were just as good as those of any other 160-lb. lifter, they fell considerably short of the records made by the giants in the lifting game. Nevertheless, he could have fairly been described as being stronger than two ordinary men.

It is very hard for the ordinary citizen to gauge the strength of a real "Strong Man." He goes to a vaudeville show to see a "Strong Act," and he watches the performer stoop under a platform on which fifteen or twenty men are standing, and lift the whole weight on his back. Mr. Ordinary Citizen has never tried this stunt, but doubts whether he could raise 500 lbs. in that way, and so concludes that this performer is many times as strong as he is. Next, he sees the performer take a big bar-bell weighing 250 lbs., and slowly push it above the head with one hand. This is a stunt that the ordinary citizen knows something about. He has probably tried and failed to put up a 50-lb. weight, so that the performer's 250-lb. lift impresses him greatly. It will probably surprise you when I tell you that the ordinary man, after a few months of the right kind of training, can develop enough strength to put up 150 lbs. with one hand, and to raise 2,000 lbs. on his back in a "platform-lift." That is enough to make you gasp; I mean you, who are reading these lines. You have always considered yourself as "just the average individual," and at first you cannot grasp the idea that it would be possible for you to learn to accomplish Herculean feats of strength. Yet I, who have seen so many "ordinary citizens" become able to do stunts of this kind, can assure you that your possibilities are, in all likelihood, just as great as those of any other average citizen.

In his book on Physical Education, Dr. Felix Oswald said that one company of soldiers in the Middle Ages would contain more "Strong Men" than would be found in a modern army corps. I cannot agree with this statement. I will admit that possibly the average man of three hundred years ago was stronger than the average man of today, because in those days there were no labor-saving devices, and practically every man had to use his muscles a great deal more than the average man of today uses his. Nevertheless, the strongest men of today are just as strong as or stronger than the "Strong Men" of three hundred years ago.

For example, I have a collection of books dealing with the subject of strength, and almost every one of these books starts off by telling you of the wonderful feats of strength accomplished by the mighty men of the past. One man, who is always mentioned, is Thomas Topham, who was born in London in 1710. When Topham was thirty-one, he made a lift of 1836 lbs. Three barrels of water were chained together. Topham stood on a platform above the barrels, and around his neck was a leather strap which was attached to a chain. This chain passed through a hole in the platform on which he was standing, and was coupled to the chain that bound the barrels together. Topham bent his legs and back slightly, and placed his hands on a couple of braces. Then, by simultaneously straightening his arms, back, and legs, he lifted the barrels a couple of inches from the ground. The writers of the books I mentioned always recite this feat as something incredible, and certainly it seems to have been sufficient to preserve Topham's name and fame as a "strong man."

One Saturday afternoon, early in 1917, I had a number of celebrated lifters come to my factory, and give an exhibition before an audience of about one hundred experts. Most of the lifting was done with bar-bells, and one or two records were created on that afternoon. In the factory we had a lifting platform (the one shown in Fig. 3). This platform, as you can see by looking at the pictures, is a double affair. The lifter stands on the upper platform, and raises the lower one. After the regular exhibition was over, one of the lifters wished to try his strength at lifting with a harness around the neck. We did not use barrels of water; but we piled 50-lb. weights on the bottom platform. This man had never attempted this lift before; so we started off with a moderate weight. After he had made a lift we would throw more weights on the bottom platform. He went as high as 2400 lbs. Neither I nor anyone else present considered that lift extraordinary. We fully expected him to lift that much, and every experienced lifter present knew that if he had practiced the lift for a few weeks, he could do 3000 lbs. When I wrote a description of the exhibition for the STRENGTH Magazine, I did not even mention that stunt; but the fact remains that this man (Adolph Nordquest) lifted 550 lbs. more than Topham did; so if Topham was the strongest man of his day, then "Strong Men" must have improved since that time.

In this book I will talk a great deal about lifters and lifting, which means that I will have to say a great deal about heavy bar-bells and dumbbells; but I do not mean you to think that I claim it is only lifters and bar-bell users who are gifted with super-strength. As a matter of fact, super-strength is not a gift of nature. If it were, there would be no use of writing this book;

because if great strength was the monopoly of a few favored individuals, what would be the use of you trying to acquire such strength? For every man who inherits great strength, or who possesses great strength by virtue of having an unusually large and powerfully made body, there are a dozen other men who have deliberately and purposely made themselves strong. I have seen laborers, farmers, football players, physicians, singers, artists and business men who were wonderfully built and tremendously strong; but every one of these men could have been improved by a course of scientific training. To balance that, I have seen scores of men and boys who started with below-average development, and very little strength, who have absolutely converted themselves into "Strong Men " All these individuals got their strength, health and development by practicing with adjustable bar-bells.

Of course, there are lots of men who are wonderfully strong who have never seen a bar-bell. I am personally acquainted with many such men; but I must say that there is not one among them whom I could not have made still stronger by putting him on a special training program with weights. On the other hand, I have never seen a man who was naturally weak get into the "Strong Man" class except by the use of weights.

There are some authorities who seem to think that it is foolish for any man to try to improve the body to any great extent; and such authorities are apt to speak in a slighting way of what they call "made" strong men. When I was younger, such remarks used to worry me; but in the last twenty years I have seen so many of these "made" strong men sweep aside the lifting-records made by the natural giants, that I have come to the conclusion that "made" strength is just as valuable and lasting as is natural, or inherited, strength.

The greatest French authority on the subject of strength is Prof. Des Bonnet. His book, "The Kings of Strength," contains a description (with pictures) of several hundred of the most celebrated "strong men" of the last seventy-five years. In the body of this book you will find pictures of men like Sandow, Arthur Saxon, Hackenschmidt, and many other celebrated athletes who are familiar to you as being among the strongest men in recent history. In the back of his book Des Bonnet has a special section devoted to two men whom he calls "super-athletes"; and these two men were Louis Cyr, of Canada, and Apollon, of France. He places them in a class by themselves.

Now, as many of you are aware, Saxon, Sandow, Hackenschmidt, and many of the other celebrated "Strong Men" are of average height; and their unusual power is due to the great size and strength of their muscles. Cyr and Apollon were giants. Cyr stood 6 feet and weighed over 300 lbs., and was built on a vastly larger mold than the average "Strong Man." Apollon stood we'll over 6 feet in height and had a tremendous frame. Undoubtedly both of these men were giants in strength as well as being giants in size; but, just the same, if we go by the records, they do not seem to have been able to deliver more strength than did some of their smaller rivals. For example, Cyr's best record in the two- arm jerk was 345 lbs., Arthur Saxon, who weighed 100 lbs. less than Cyr, also did 345 lbs. in that particular lift. It is true that Cyr lifted the bell in one motion from the floor to the chest, before tossing it to arms' length above his head; whereas Saxon had to raise the bell in two movements to his chest. Nevertheless, he raised it just as much above his head as Cyr did. Two years ago I saw Henry Steinborn, who is only a little bit heavier than Saxon, raise in one motion to the chest, and then jerk aloft with both arms, a bar-bell weighing 347 lbs.; thereby beating Cyr's record. A few nights later some friends of mine saw Steinborn raise 375 lbs. in the same style.

Again, Cyr's best record in the one-arm press is 273 lbs.; and that mark has been beaten by a dozen smaller men. I admit that these men use a style which is different from the method Cyr used; but it can't be denied that some of these men have beaten Cyr's record by anywhere from 20 to 50 lbs.; and in the one-arm press the palm goes to the man who can put up the most weight. Cyr, unquestionably, had bigger muscles and a bigger frame and more natural strength than most lifters have; but he could not exert that strength to much advantage, except when he was in certain positions.

The bodily strength possessed by the so-called "Strong Men," whether amateur or professional, is vastly greater than the strength possessed by the average gymnast, track athlete, oarsman, football player, or workman. The "Strong Man" has a different kind of strength. His arms may be no bigger than those of a Roman-ring performer; his legs may be no bigger than those of a great football player; but he has a bodily strength which is not possessed by any other class of athlete; and this bodily strength is due, first, to the perfect development of every muscle, and, second, to the ability of making those muscles co-ordinate. As I go on writing these chapters, I intend to continually hammer away in an endeavor to "put over" this idea of bodily strength, as contrasted to arm strength. For most of you, I know, have the fixed idea that a "Strong Man" is strong only because he has such wonderful arms.

Let me tell you another story: this time about an amateur. This man was walking with three companions, when they came to a gate in a high, iron fence. The amateur "Strong Man" slipped through the gate; slammed it shut; and then invited his three friends to open it. He stretched his arms straight out in front of him, and with each hand grasping one of the upright iron rods in the gate, leaned forward and braced himself in the position shown in the illustration (Fig. 9). After a terrific struggle, which lasted a couple of minutes, the other three men succeeded in pushing the gate open; but they did not push the athlete over backwards. He kept himself in the same position, although his feet gradually slipped backwards. It was only his extraordinary bodily strength which enabled him to exert as much pressure against one side of the gate as his three friends combined could exert against the other side. His arms did very little of the work; they were held rigidly straight, and merely transmitted the pressure exerted by the flexed muscles of his legs and body. On top of that, he applied his strength scientifically. If he had arched his back, or straightened the advanced leg, he would soon have been toppled over backwards. Here is another man who may not have been as strong as three ordinary men; but he certainly was as strong as two.

I could tell you a dozen other such stories; as, for example, how Cyr leaned his mighty shoulders against the end of a loaded freight car and, walking backwards, pushed that car up a slight grade, a stunt in which the arms were not used at all. How other athletes managed to lift hundreds, and even thousands of pounds by the strength of their legs; but I will bring those stories in where they belong.

CHAPTER II

THE BACK

The keystone of the arch of a man's strength is the "small" of his back. A man may have wonderful arms and fair legs; but if he is weak in the loins and in the lower part of the back, he can never be classed as a real "Strong Man." Gymnasts and trapeze performers frequently have wonderful arms and shoulders. Some of the vaudeville artists, who specialize on Roman-ring work, are noted for their arm development. Some of them can take hold of a swinging ring with the right hand, and "chin" themselves several times in succession; but almost all of these men have small legs and puny hips. Lightness of weight in the lower half of the body is a positive advantage to a man who earns his living as a professional gymnast; because the smaller and lighter his legs are, the easier it is for him to do stunts on a trapeze or a pair of Roman rings. But put that man in a big packing establishment where he would be required to carry a half-carcass of beef on one shoulder; or in the line of a varsity football team, and his big arm muscles would be but little good to him. I mention this because there are some physical culturists who cling to the idea that "chinning" the horizontal bar, and "dipping" on the parallel bars, is the kind of work which best prepares a man for weight-lifting. According to my experience, it is easier to make a great lifter out of a man who has powerful legs, a strong back and but moderate arms; than a man who has big arms and poor under-pinning. Most ground-tumblers could easily become high-grade strong men; because performing such stunts as turning handsprings, cartwheels and somersaults creates far more bodily strength than one can get by doing arm-stunts on the horizontal and the parallel bars. I once witnessed a friendly tussle between a tumbler and a gymnast.

Both men weighed about the same; the gymnast had 15-inch arms and 20-inch thighs; whereas the tumbler had 14-inch arms and 22½-inch thighs. When they came together, the tumbler took hold of the gymnast and ran him backwards across the gym; and then up-ended him and stood him on his head. The tumbler's constant springing, leaping, bending and twisting had given him great strength in the thighs and waist; and that is the kind of strength which enables a man to push forward against great resistance, and to keep his feet against the onslaught of a powerful opponent.

It may surprise you to know that only a strong-backed man can lift great weights to arms' length above the head. One of the simplest training stunts of the lifters is to take a bar-bell in both hands and push it several times in succession to arms'-length above the head. A man who is accustomed to using bar-bells will do this quickly and easily; and when he pushes the bell aloft his body will remain erect. Anyone who had never used weights, on seeing a lifter raise the bar-bell in this easy fashion, would be apt to exclaim, "My! that chap must have strong arms to be able to push up a heavy weight in that way." If the lifter invited the bystander to try to push the bell aloft, here is what would probably happen: In the first place, the novice would have considerable difficulty in raising the 100-lb. bell from the floor to the chest, on account of the lack of strength in his back; and if he did get it to the shoulder he might press it to arms' length; but, as he did so, his body would be bent over backwards at the waist-line, he would have to make a tremendous effort, would get red in the face and, after he had lowered the bell to the ground, would probably complain that he had wrenched the small of his back.

The above is not a supposititious case. It is a thing that I have seen happen dozens of times, even when the novice at weight-lifting was a man who had spent months, or even years, at light exercises. I have seen gymnasts with fine upper arms (which they had developed through chinning the bar and dipping on the horizontal bars)fail to press aloft a weight so light that it would be a joke to the average lifter. In such cases, the gymnast is usually quite puzzled. He knows that his arms are as big as are the lifter's arms, and he thinks that he has failed because he has not the "knack" of lifting; whereas, the reason for his failure is merely lack of back strength. Here is one thing that you, who read this book, must get firmly fixed in your mind; and that is, when a man is standing on his feet he positively cannot exert the full strength of his arms unless the strength of his back and legs is in proportion to the strength of his arms. I do not mean that the back must be just as strong as the arms, but that it must be many times stronger.

I understand that in these college "strength tests," when they wish to get a record of a student's back-strength, they put a leather collar around his neck, have him stand with legs straight, lean forward from the hips, and then attempt to bring his body to the upright position. The collar referred to is a loop of strap attached to a chain; which, in turn, is attached to some spring registering device. After this test is completed the student is told to stand with his body upright, his legs slightly bent, and then to endeavor to straighten the legs so as to get a register of his leg-strength.

I find that it is almost impossible to disassociate the strength of the legs and back. In the back test referred to above it might seem to you that, in the act of bringing the body to the upright position, the student would use only his back muscles; but, as a matter of fact, he also uses most of the muscles of the haunches and those on the back of the thighs. When you stand with the legs stiff and straight and bend the body over, the hips are the joint which form the hinge. Supposing you wished to hang a very heavy door, you would naturally buy a pair of heavy hinges; but, of course, the leaf of the hinge which fastened to the door would be no thicker nor heavier than the leaf which fastened to the door-frame. You would not think of picking out a pair of hinges with leaves of different thickness. Even if the leaf which fastened to the door were a quarter of an inch thick, you would know that the hinge would be no good if the leaf which fastened to the door-frame was made of tin and only one- sixteenth of an inch thick. When you lean over in the manner described and pull against a registering machine, or pick up a heavy weight, your back corresponds to that part of the hinge which is fastened to the door, and your legs to that part which is fastened to the door-frame. Therefore, unless his legs are powerfully developed, no man can show a high record in a test of back-strength. In fact, as we go along, you will become more and more impressed with this interdependence of the muscles. You will find that in any feat of super-strength the athlete who accomplishes it uses as many muscles as possible. The reason that so many strength records were made, and are held, by men who have practiced with weights, is because when a man uses weights he is practically compelled to use his muscles in interlocking groups.

In this chapter, when I refer to the back, I particularly mean the muscles in the back which control the action of the spine. On either side of the spine there are long muscles which run all the way from the base of the skull to the hips; and these muscles are called the "erector spinae"; that is, the muscles which straighten or erect the spine. In the lower half of the back, these muscles are plainly visible, and when fully developed they appear like two ships'- cables. If you wish to gauge the strength of a man's back don't look at his shoulders, but at the small of his back—his loins, his haunches and the back of his thighs.

If you were to embark on a program of exercise to improve your body, and if you happened to select some system of light exercise, you would find that there were a great many of those exercises in which you held in each hand a moderate weight and did motions to increase the development of the arms, the shoulders and the muscles on the upper part of the trunk. You would get comparatively few exercises for the lower part of the back and for the legs; and it is likely that you would be told that merely bending (and doing other movements which compelled you to raise the weight of your own body) would be sufficient to develop the back muscles to their full extent.

Now this is very far from being true. The lower back muscles are prodigiously powerful when fully developed; and it takes more than raising the weight of your own body to bring out that full development. The simplest of all exercises for developing the muscles which control the spine, is the one in which you stand with the legs stiff and straight, and then bend the body over by arching the spine, and touch the floor with the tips of your fingers. When you bend over, all you do is to stretch the muscles along the spine and the back of the legs. It is contraction, and not stretching, which develops muscles; so that these muscles do their real work as your body is raised again to the upright position. Yet nine men out of ten think that the important part of the exercise is the bending over. (In fact, most people use this exercise to reduce the size of the abdomen.) In order to get any noticeable development of the back, it would be necessary to repeat that exercise several hundred times in succession; whereas, if you put a further tax on the back muscles, by holding a moderate amount of weight in your hands, you can, by making a couple of dozen repetitions, develop back muscles of much larger size and very much higher quality.

The proper way to perform this exercise is shown in Fig. 10. The beginner of average size should use 20 or 30 lbs., and after he can use that weight without perceptible exertion he should add 5 or 10 lbs. more, gradually working up to about 75 lbs. A big man can safely start with 40 or 50 lbs. and can go as high as 100 lbs. as an exercising weight. This is not a lift or a feat of strength; neither is it the correct way to raise very heavy weights from the ground. It is just an exercise; but, by keeping the legs stiff and straight, and doing all the bending by arching the spine, you can get a remarkable pair of "erector-spinae" muscles. To those of you who have never had a weight in your hands the idea of "exercising" with a 100-lb. weight seems almost fantastic. That is just because you have not even the faintest conception of the possibilities of your own body. To do this exercise with 25 or

30 lbs. is no harder than carrying a scuttle of coal up one flight of stairs, and most of you can do that without trouble. Continued practice of the foregoing movement for a few weeks will so develop the back muscles that you can then use 80 or 100 lbs. with no more exertion than was necessary when you were using 30 lbs. Furthermore, you will find that when you use 100 lbs. this exercise will have the most surprising effect on the way you walk. Where you had formerly gone upstairs one step at a time, you would now find yourself going up two or three steps at a time, just for the pure joy of it; and if you could stand between the big triplicate mirrors (such as the tailors use) you would find that, along the small of the back, you had two big cables of muscle, such as those shown in Fig. 6.

In some systems of exercise, instead of merely bending over and touching the floor with finger tips, you are told to stand stiff-legged, with the feet spread apart, and then to take a light dumbbell in each hand, bend forward, swing the bells backwards between the legs, and then swing them to arms'-length overhead. This is a better exercise than touching the floor, because the light bells are swung backwards at arms'-length; and this movement, on account of the increase in the leverage, gives fairly vigorous exercise to the back muscles, even when a pair of light bells is used. But that is just another spine exercise. If you wish to get super-strength it is absolutely necessary for you to teach your back to work in concert with the legs. Later on, in the chapter about dead-weight lifting, I will show you how many so-called "back-lifts" are really "back-and-leg" lifts, in which the legs do most of the work.

Every great "Strong Man," whether amateur or professional, has had to master the secret of the "flat back," which is one of the most vital requisites of super-strength. The description of the positions in which a "Strong Man" uses the "flat back" belongs just as much in the chapter about the legs as it belongs here, but we may as well have it now. The main point to be remembered is that any individual, athlete or otherwise, can deliver several times as much power when his back is flat and his spine straight, as he can when his spine is arched. This applies in practically any feat of weight-lifting, or actual labor, where it is necessary to move, shift, lift, or carry an article weighing several hundred pounds. When a truckman or porter wants to move or up-end a square case containing, say, 1000 lbs. of material, he does not stand close to it and push with bent arms and arched spine. He stands at arms'-length, rests his hands against some part of the case, keeps his arms straight and his back flat, and does all pushing with his legs, as in Fig. 9. In that position he is able to employ the full strength of his back.

About the best exercise for strengthening the back and legs, and for teaching them to work together, is the one shown in Figs. 12 and 13. It takes considerable practice to master it; but it is worth all the trouble, because it is one of the fundamentals of super- strength. You stand with the feet about 16 inches apart and strongly braced, and then take a kettle-bell and swing it backwards between the legs, as in Fig. 12. As the kettle-bell goes backwards you bend your legs slightly at the knees, and lean the body forward from the hips; but you must not arch the spine. (In Fig. 12 you will see that the back of the athlete is almost as flat as a board.) From this position you swing the bell forward; and, as you do so, you bring the body to an upright position. This will make the kettle-bell swing at arms'-length straight in front of you and at about the height of your chest, as in Fig. 13. At that exact second you must release the kettle-bell with the right hand, grasp it with the left, and swung it back again. After each swing you must change hands and, as you bend over, you rest the free hand on the knee.

Start this exercise with a kettle-bell weighing 20 or 25 lbs., and learn to do the movement smoothly and easily. At first, you will be inclined to fumble when you change hands. I have seen beginners try to slowly and painstakingly shift the bell from one hand to the other. The right way is to open the fingers of the lifting hand and let the bell start to fly away from you, and then to grab it with the other hand before it has had time to travel even an inch forwards. After a few days' practice you will get so that you can change the weight from one hand to the other at the top of the swing, without the slightest interruption of the rhythm of the swinging movement. As soon as you have mastered the movement, commence to add weight to your kettle-bell. It will not be many weeks before you can use a 75-lb. kettle-bell in this way, and not long after that before you can handle 100 lbs.

This exercise has so many beneficial effects that it should be included in the training of everyone who aspires to super-strength. If you keep your back flat there is not the least danger of hurting yourself. Since your whole attention is concentrated on the swinging of the kettle-bell it is impossible for you to see whether you are doing it correctly; and so you should have a friend watch you and tell you whether you are keeping your back flat. Do not be so anxious to keep the back flat that you go to the other extreme and make the back hollow. The whole idea is to keep the spine as straight as possible and to do all the bending with the hips and knees.

Here are a few of the things you will gain from this exercise: You will learn to instinctively keep your back flat when making a great exertion; you will get a much firmer grip on the ground with your feet; you will learn how to "time" a heavy moving object; you will increase the gripping power of the hands and increase the development of the front part of the shoulder muscles; you will become able to jump further and higher. It is because "Strong Men" practice such exercises as this, that they are able to make such remarkable records in the standing broad-jump and standing high-jump. I know a lifter 40 years old and weighing 220 lbs. who can clear almost eleven feet in a standing broad-jump. At the age of twenty-five, when he was lifting professionally, he could jump even further than that; and, what is more, he could sprint 100 yards in 10 seconds flat. Incidentally, he holds one or two records in lifting heavy weights from the ground.

In the last chapter you will find some remarks concerning the influence which lower-back development has upon a man's vitality and virility.

CHAPTER III

SOME LIFTING RECORDS

When I first became interested in bar-bells I collected a lot of data about weight-lifting records. There was a time when I could tell you the world's record in almost any lift you could mention. I could tell you the records for the best men in the different nations at the same lift. I knew the name of the man who made the record, when he made it, exactly how many pounds he lifted, and which other men had come closest to equaling his record. As I grow older I find that I care less and less about records and more and more about body-building. It seems to me to be much more important to help a man to get a finely proportioned body, great muscular and organic vigor, and a higher degree of development, than to set him at record making. Since my interests have changed, my stock of information about records has grown less and less. As you go on you will undoubtedly notice that many a time I will tell you a record is "about" so and so; and that means that I am not sure whether any new records have been made abroad since 1914. I could start and give you lifting records, some of which would be exact and some approximate; but unless you happen to be a skilled lifter, such records would mean nothing to you. In this chapter I am going to tell you most of the records in back-and-leg lifting, and, as you read along, you will find chapters telling you how to develop certain parts of the body, followed by other chapters giving you the records in lifts where the athlete uses the muscles described in the preceding chapter.

Possibly the most common test of strength in all the world is to lean the body over, take hold of a heavy weight, and raise it from the ground. In weight-lifting circles this is known as the "dead-weight" lift or "hands-alone." It is exactly such a lift as a lot of powerful laborers or porters would naturally select if they wished to determine which the strongest man among them was. When a bar-bell is used the lift is performed as follows: The lifter first stands with his heels together and the handle of the bell over his insteps; then he leans over, by bending a little at the knees and a good deal at the hips, and grasps the bar-bell with both hands, as in Fig. 14, the palm of one hand being forward, and the knuckles of the other hand forward; then he straightens up (that is, stands erect), bringing the bar-bell with him, as in Fig. 15. Since the knees are bent only slightly it is necessary to arch the spine and curve the back in order to reach down and get hold of the bar-bell handle. Therefore, it is not possible to lift very much weight in this way. The English amateur record is 533 lbs.; but Mr. Jowett says that he has seen a 140-lb. Canadian lifter raise 500 lbs., and that he saw a gigantic Canadian, Lavallee, perform the lift with 800 lbs. I have seen several men raise between 550 and 600 lbs. in this way, but they did not stand with the heels together as in the English style. I, personally, cannot see any reason for standing in that way. If the lifter were to stand with the feet about 8 inches apart he would be much more firmly braced and could exert considerably more strength. This is a lift which any unskilled man can perform, and it is a fairly good test of the natural strength of the back. A big, 200-lb. truck driver, or one of the Herculean lumbermen from our

Western states, could probably do 400 lbs. in this lift the first time he tried it, because his work has been just along this line, and the years he has spent in the daily handling of heavy logs and heavy cases of goods have developed the muscles used in the lift. On the other hand, a gymnast, or a business man whose greatest physical exertion is practicing bending movements, would probably be "stopped" with a 250-lb. bar-bell. Therefore, if you are not used to heavy work or vigorous exercise, do not make the mistake of starting to practice the dead-weight lift with 300 to 350 lbs. That would be just as foolish as for a non-swimmer to jump off a ferryboat in mid-river. But if you practice the two back exercises described in the preceding chapter, then, when you have gotten so that you can handle 100 lbs. in those exercises, you will find you can outdo the average truck driver or lumberman in dead-weight lifting.

At noon hour, on one day several years ago, I went into my factory and I found a number of lifters competing at the dead-weight lift. Some of the competitors were customers, and others were the men who made bar-bells; and every one of them were accustomed to handling heavy weights. I asked them why they didn't try the "hand-and-thigh" lift, and found, to my surprise, that they were unacquainted with that style; so, naturally, I demonstrated it to them and lifted two or three hundred pounds more than they had been using. That was not because I was very strong, but because I was using a much easier style.

A week later, when I went into the factory, several of these same men made "hand-and-thigh" lifts with three or four hundred pounds more than I had lifted. It had taken them only one look to grasp the principle of the style, and they had put in a little quiet practice. This was so interesting to me that I immediately ordered the lifting platform shown in Fig. 3. If you examine the picture you will notice that the weights to be lifted are placed on the lower platform, and that from the superstructure of this lower platform there is a rod which projects vertically upward through a hole in the upper platform. The upper end of this rod was threaded so that the lifting-handle could be screwed up or down, so as to suit the height of the lifter. In making a "hand-and- thigh" lift, the athlete would adjust his handle so that when he bent his knees the handle would come just to the top of the thighs, as shown in Fig. 17. He would then take hold of the handle bar allowing his knuckles to rest against the thighs. When lifting the weight he would lean a trifle backwards and straighten the legs.

When making a lift like this, all one has to do is to get the weight clear of the ground; but sometimes the lifter is deceived because he thinks he has raised the lower platform, when he has only titled it and raised one end of it from the ground. So we rigged up an electric connection at each end of the lower platform, and when the platform was lifted fairly and squarely for one- quarter of an inch, a circuit was completed and a bell rang. If only one end of the platform were lifted the bell did not ring.

In this lift the greater part of the work is done by the legs. When a very heavy weight was used, the lifter's knuckles were forced into the flesh of his thigh, making it necessary to throw a pad across the upper legs. By placing the hands on the thighs in this way the force with which he could grip the bar was greatly increased. No one ever complained that he could feel the strain in the legs, although almost every one noticed that the effort of pulling with the hands produced a perceptibly dragging effect on the trapezius muscles, which lift the shoulders. (Some of the men found that they could add 100 or 200 lbs. to their record by leaning further back, thus supplementing the strength of the legs with the strength of the back muscles.) I understand that the world's record in this lift is about 1850 lbs. The men who used our platform were not back-lifters nor harness-lifters, but bar-bell lifters; consequently, after the first novelty had worn off, the platform was rarely used. Nevertheless, I saw some of these bar-bell lifters (men who weighed 160 to 175 lbs.) raise over 1200 lbs., and one or two of them went as high as 1500 lbs. If they had taken the trouble to prepare themselves for the lift by practicing leg exercises, they might have gone as high as 1600 lbs. Some of the giants, like Cyr, Barre and Travis, could probably have gone close to the record, or even beaten it. My experience was that any fair bar-bell lifter could raise over 1000 lbs. within a day or two after he had mastered the principle of the lift.

Just below the bar-bell factory was the garage of a piano-moving concern which employed a lot of big, husky workmen. Some one told these men about the lifting-platform, and one day a half dozen of them came in to try this lift. There was not one among them who weighed less than 180 lbs., and some of them must have weighed 220. They were the typical broad-shouldered, wide- backed, thick-legged type whom you would expect to see carrying pianos up flights of stairs. Not one of these men was able to lift 800 lbs. in the hand-and-thigh style; and they never came back to try again, because one of our chaps, who weighed only 165 lbs., raised 1250 lbs. on that occasion. Nevertheless, I believe that almost any one of these visitors could have raised almost as much if he had practiced for a week or so, because the very nature of their daily work developed the muscles used in this lift.

Another form of dead-weight lifting is the so-called "Jefferson Lift," evidently named for the old-time lifter. In this style it is customary to use a pear-shaped or pyramidal weight, surmounted by a crossbar at about 24 inches from the ground. We had no such weight, so we used a bar-bell. The lifter straddles the bar, with one hand in front of it and the other behind it, and the palms of the hands facing each other, as in Fig. 18. I can't tell you the record in this lift, but it is not nearly as high as in the hand-and- thigh style, because the strain on the hands is so great that the fingers are apt to be pulled out straight. Also the strain on the shoulders is very much greater, as they are pulled down forcibly in the act of raising the weight from the floor. You should note that while the lifter inclines his body slightly forward from the hips that, nevertheless, he keeps his spine straight, and that most of the work is done by the act of straightening the legs. In such lifts the arms are merely connecting rods or links. No man could raise a big weight in the Jefferson Style with his arms bent.

PLATE 1

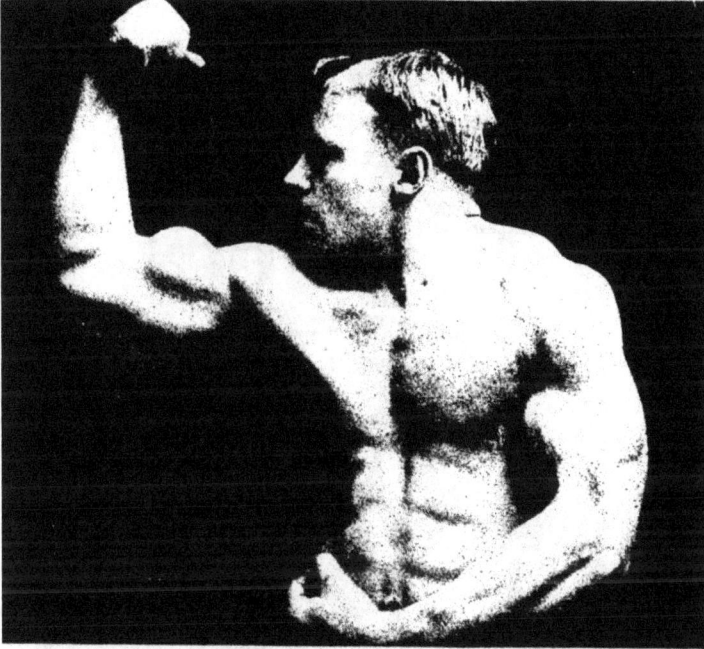

Fig. 1

Plate 1, Figures 1 and 2. Charles Herold, the middle-weight "Strong Man"; who is the athlete referred to in the first part of the first chapter

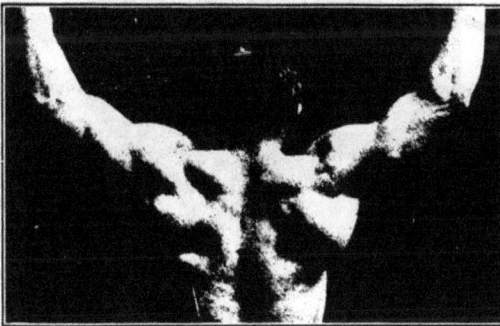

Fig. 2

PLATE 2

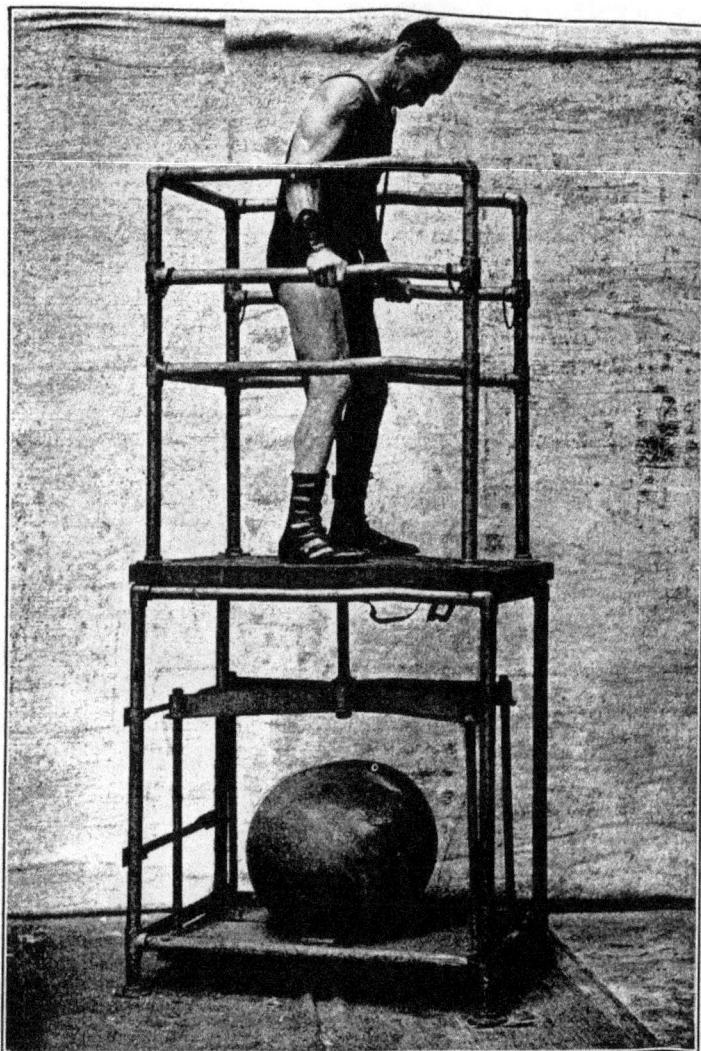

Fig. 3
Plate 2, Figure 3. Walter Donald demonstrating the "Harness Lift". In this style of harness, a loop of leather passes over each shoulder. The weight used is a trifle—only about 600 lbs.

PLATE 3

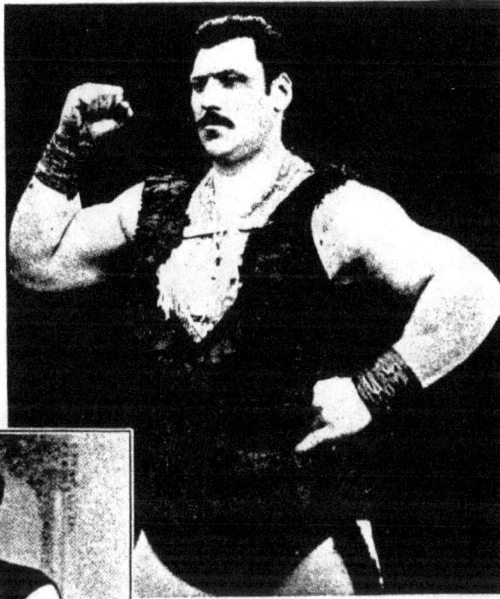

Fig. 4

late 3, Figure 4.
pollon, the giant
ench lifter, cred-
ed by Prof. Des
onnett as being one
the two strongest
en in the world.
is right forearm
easured 16 inches
hen the arm was
raight, and 19
ches when in the
osition shown in
this picture

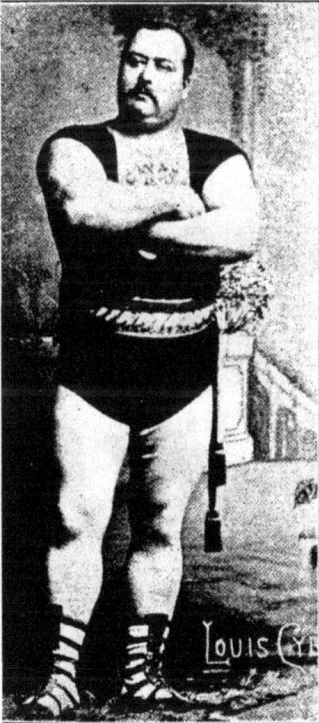

Fig. 5

Figure 5. The famous Louis
Cyr, of Canada, whose
strength has become a tradition. Apollon and Cyr were
undoubtedly the two strongest men of their time, and
both of them were natural
giants. Most of their records
have been eclipsed by
smaller, though more active,
modern lifters

31

PLATE 4

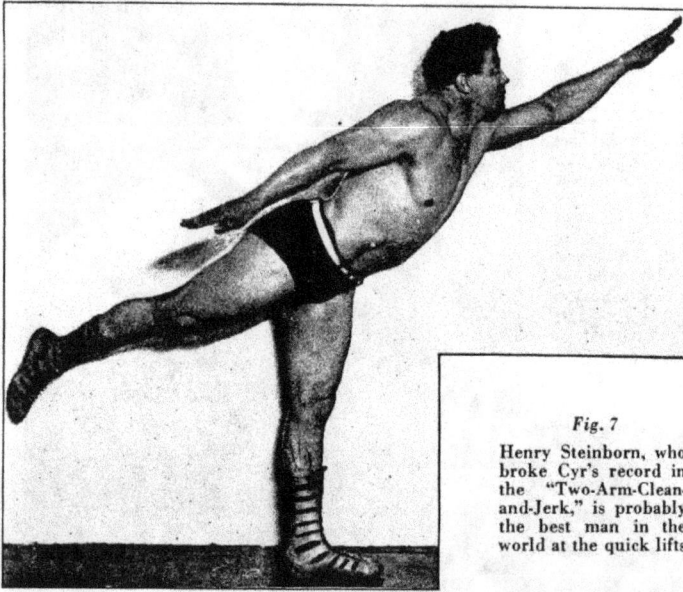

Fig. 7

Henry Steinborn, who broke Cyr's record in the "Two-Arm-Clean-and-Jerk," is probably the best man in the world at the quick lifts

Fig. 6

Plate 4, Figure 6. Adolph Nordquest, who made the "Harness Lift" referred to in the first chapter. Note the tremendous size and development of the muscles on either side of the spine

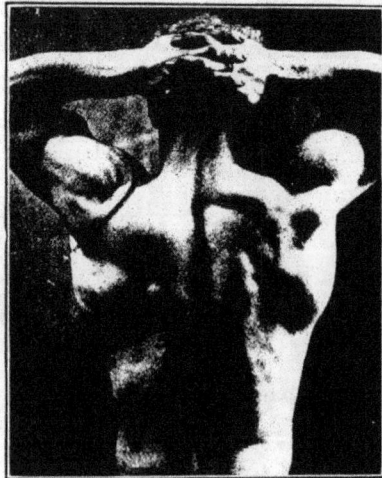

PLATE 5

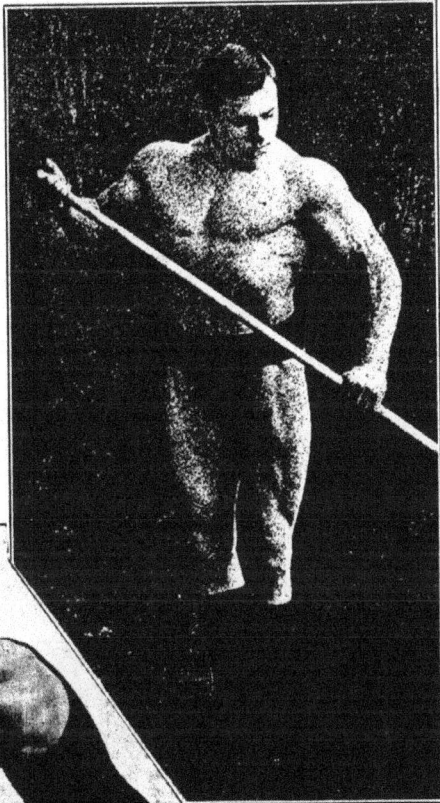

Fig. 8

Plate 5, Figure 8. George Hackenschmidt in a pose which reveals the great breadth of his shoulders and the enormous size of his chest

Fig 9

Figure 9. Showing the position in which a man can exert the greatest strength in p u s h i n g forward

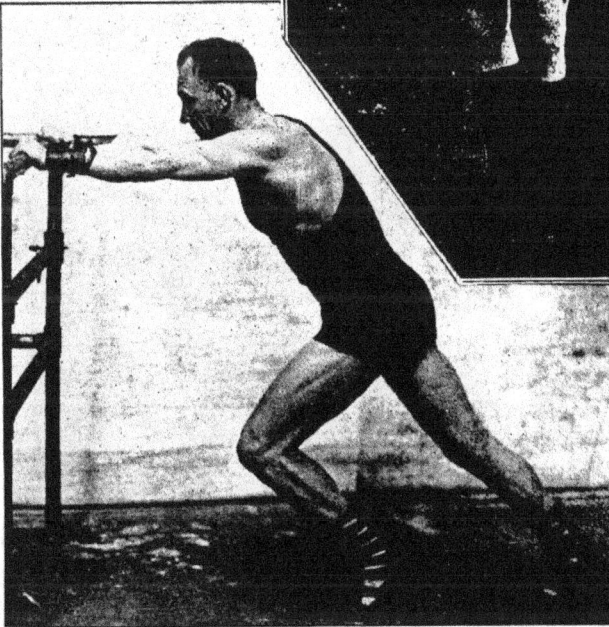

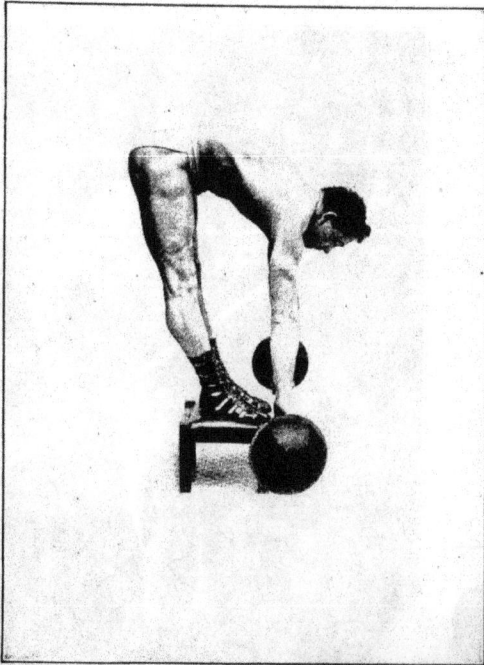

PLATE 6

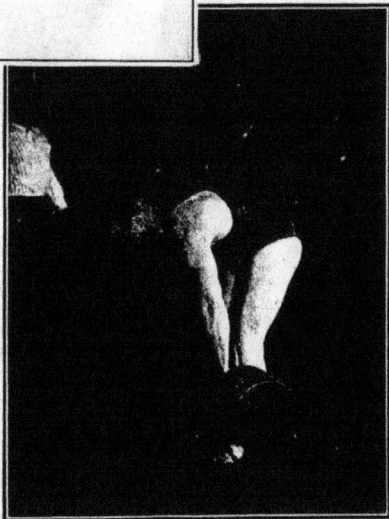

Fig. 10

Plate 6, Figure 10. An exercise to develop the muscles which r u n a l o n g either side of the spine, and which do most of the work in lifting a heavy weight f r o m the ground. This exercise can be made more effective if you stand on a box, or pile of books, as this will enable you to bend further over.

Fig. 11

Figure 11. Adolph Nordquest m a k i n g a "Dead Weight Lift" with 638 lbs. The muscles used in this lift are developed by practicing the exercise shown in Figure 10. When doing the exercise, you should keep the legs straight and stiff. In making the lift, you are allowed to bend the legs slightly at the knees.

CHAPTER IV

THE LEGS

The man who exercises in his own room with a pair of light dumbbells, who uses a pair of pulley-weights, or swings a pair of wooden Indian clubs, rarely gets even acquainted with the immense power which is lying dormant in his back and legs. As I said before, mere bending movements will never develop the back or waist muscles to their full size; neither will the ordinary leg-exercises produce a really powerful pair of lower limbs. A bar-bell so heavy that you could not possibly raise it by the strength of the unassisted arm muscles, is a mere plaything for the leg muscles. Take, for example, the lifter mentioned in the story which opens the first chapter. This man could take a 220-lb. bar-bell in both hands, raise it from the floor to the shoulders and, without leaning backwards, slowly press the bar-bell to arms' length above the head. In this lift, which is called the "military press," the work of elevating the bell is done by the extensor muscles of the arms and the muscles on the points of the shoulders. I once saw this same man lie flat on his back and hold on the soles of his up-raised feet, a plank bearing twelve men; a total weight of more than 1600 lbs. After he had the weight securely balanced, he would allow his legs to bend slightly at the knees, thus lowering the plank three or four inches, and then would push the weight up again by the sheer strength of his leg muscles.

The hardest part of any "pressing" is the start. This man might have taken a 300-lb. bar-bell and raised it to arms' length by what is known as the "two-arm jerk," and then have lowered it 4 inches by bending the arms, and pressed it again to arms' length; but even then the pressing power in his arms was less than one-fifth the pressing power in his legs. I am sorry that I can't show you a full-length picture, but I can assure you that his legs were just as well developed as his arms, which are shown in Figs. 1 and 2. I have seen this man lie flat on his back, lift a 200-lb. barbell with his hands, place it on the soles of his feet, as in Fig. 20, and then press it up to the full stretch of his legs two hundred times in succession. Every time he bent his legs he brought his knees down until they almost touched his chest, and every time he raised the bell he was particular to get the legs perfectly straight. He practiced bare-footed, and balanced the bell on the balls of the feet; but if you try it you'd better wear a pair of ordinary street shoes, and let the handle of the bell rest against the projecting heels. When you first attempt it you will have some difficulty in placing the bell on the soles of your feet, particularly if you happen to be stout; because the knees have to be pressed against the chest in order to get the feet so low that you can reach up with the hands and place the bell in position. I advise you to start with not more than 25 lbs., making quite a number of repetitions, and then to increase the weight so often as you comfortably can. This exercise develops most of the muscles in the thighs, and it seems to have a peculiar effect in developing the biceps muscles on the back of the thigh; but you will not get such development if you fail to press the legs to full stretch every time you raise the bell. I once saw in vaudeville a "Strong Man" named Carl Victor, from Pittsburgh. He used several variations of this stunt in his act, and you could see that it was a favorite exercise of his. He had a magnificent pair of legs and probably the best development on the back, or under side, of the thigh, that I have ever seen.

Now, exactly reverse this stunt. When you lie flat on the back your hips are pressed against the floor, and the weight is raised on the feet. If you stand on your feet and life a very heavy weight by a chain which is attached to a belt around the hips, as in Fig. 21, you use almost the same muscles that you do in the preceding stunt. The picture of Mr. Roy L. Smith, Fig. 22, shows the way in which a "hip lift" is accomplished. Mr. Smith is shown just before he made the lift. When he straightened his legs he raised the axle and car wheels 1 inch from the ground, and the total weight lifted was 2250 lbs. Undoubtedly, Mr. Smith could lie on the back and raise, or support, that amount of weight on the soles of his feet. Mr. Smith's enormous leg strength is due to the practice of the leg exercises described in this chapter. Perhaps his favorite is a modification of the Jefferson Lift (shown in Fig. 23). In this exercise a man stands with his feet well apart and well braced, holds the bar-bell between his legs and allows it to hang at the full length of his arms. When he bends his legs he does not go any further down than shown in Fig. 23, and he keeps flat-footed. Mr. Smith will repeat this exercise a dozen times with a 300 or 350-lb. bar-bell; but the average man should start with 50 or 75 lbs.; and he should remember that all the bending is done with the legs, and that the spine must be kept straight and the body erect. In doing this exercise you positively do not lean the body forward from the hips.

An equally good, or even better, exercise would be to raise a very heavy bell by a modification of the hand-and-thigh lift. Place a heavy bar-bell on the floor in front of you; tie the ends of two ropes around the handle and the other ends around the short handle bar from your outfit. The ropes should be so short that in order to place the knuckles in the bend of the thighs you have to bend the legs about as shown in Fig. 16. Now straighten the legs and raise the weight from the floor and repeat several times. This is much easier for most people than the Jefferson Lift, or the exercise shown in Fig. 23; because when you do the Jefferson style the fingers which grip the bell will tire long before the leg muscles tire. Do not be frightened if I tell you that it is perfectly safe to start this exercise with 200 lbs.; and that after you have been practicing a few weeks you will be able to raise 500 or 600 lbs. several times in succession. If you follow the rules given there is not the slightest danger of injuring yourself or of

37

overstraining yourself. A man who has never seen a dumbbell bigger than the pairs of 5 pounders which decorate the ordinary gym, is apt to be startled if he is told to use 200 lbs. Of course, no one but an experienced man could use 200 lbs. in arm exercises, but leg exercises are an entirely different matter; and it is not until after you have practiced the two foregoing exercises that you will realize how it is that these professional "Strong Men" are able to lift, support, or carry weights which run up into the thousands of pounds. If you use bar-bells as they should be used; that is, as a means of getting magnificent body and super-strength, there is no need for you to ever perform these vaudeville stunts; but, just the same, it is a nice thing for you to feel that you could do them if you wanted to.

I have already said that a muscle exerts its greatest strength just before the point of full contraction. That is why it is safe to use weights running from 200 to 1000, or even 2000 lbs., when the legs have been bent only a trifle at the knees. When you bend the legs all the way and perform the full squat or deep knee bend, you must use a much lighter weight than in the "Jefferson" or "hand-and-thigh" exercises. The best known of all leg-developing movements is the ordinary squat, in which the athlete keeps the body erect and sits on his heels by bending the legs at the knees. If you depend just on raising the weight of your own body you will waste a lot of time in bringing the thigh muscles to the greatest development of which they are capable. There are cases where men have repeated this exercise (without weights) 2500 times without stopping; and I have seen pictures of the men who did it. Some of them had finely shaped legs of evident power; others had legs which were stringy as the limbs of a long-distance runner. Doing the deep knee bend without weights is an endurance exercise, while doing it with weights is a strength exercise. Just the same, no one should use weights until he can perform the deep knee bend fifty times in succession without weights. In order to perform the exercise correctly it is necessary to cultivate your sense of balance. I have seen beginners who could raise 350 lbs. with perfect ease in a hand-and-thigh lift, who could not repeat the deep knee bend without weights five times without losing their balance and sprawling all over the floor. If, after a test, you find that the ordinary squat is easy for you, then place a 35-lb. bar-bell on the shoulders and repeat the squat a few times, as in Fig. 24. Stand erect with the heels together, toes pointed out. As the legs are bent point the knees as far apart as possible. Then hold the bell behind you, as shown in Fig. 25. This time stand with the feet together and parallel to each other and, as you squat, point the knees directly forward. Then stand with the heels about 20 inches apart, hold the bar-bell as shown in Fig. 26 and squat flat-footed. In the first two variations you allow the heels to rise from the ground as you bend the legs. In the third variation you must keep the heels on the ground and push the knees forward and outward. The first variation develops the muscles on the outside of the thighs; the second, the muscles on the front of the thighs and right above the knees; while the third develops the muscles on the upper inside of the thighs and gives special work to the muscles of the shins.

If you start the above exercises with 25 lbs., in a few weeks you will be able to do them just as easily with 75 lbs., by reason of the increased size and strength of the thighs. Positively 40 repetitions with 75 lbs. is equivalent to 400 repetitions without a weight. You could do 120 squats altogether, 40 of each variation, and be through the work in five minutes; and you would finish up with a great feeling of springiness in the legs. If you tried to make 1000, 1500, or even 2000 repetitions without weight, it would take you the best part of half an hour and you would be as tired as though you had taken a 15-mile walk.

Leg-power and lung-power always go together. The proper way to increase the size and capacity of the lungs is not to do those arm calisthenics which are said to "open-out" the chest; but to specialize on exercises which afford vigorous work for the thighs. When doing the deep knee bend with a weight on the shoulder you should stop when the breathing becomes labored and rest a moment before starting the next exercise. For the ordinary man 150 lbs. is sufficient to bring out the full development of the muscles; and, naturally, the more weight you are using the fewer repetitions you have to make. Henry Steinborn used 400 lbs. and squatted only a half dozen times. In using very heavy weights you have to keep flat-footed, as Steinborn is doing in Fig. 27, which, by the way, shows him when half-way down. At the completion of his squat his haunches would almost touch the floor. On one occasion I saw him do the squat with 500 lbs. on his shoulders.

If a man who desired to acquire super-strength came to me and told me that he could spare only three hours a week for his exercises, I would make him spend two of these hours on leg and back exercises, and the other hour on arm and shoulder exercises for the upper body. Back and leg strength is the foundation of the so-called "abnormal" power of professional "Strong Men"; and if you who read this book are sincere in your desire to become very strong, you must never make the mistake of spending most of your time at exercises which strengthen only the arm muscles. By cultivating your back and legs you can get a fund of vitality, and a degree of bodily strength which you will never be able to get from "biceps" exercises.

I have found that while the general public seems to greatly admire the scientific lifts of a Sandow or a Hackenschmidt, it never seems anxious to emulate such lifts. On the other hand, the average man really appreciates what he calls "rough-and- ready" strength, and loudly proclaims that he prefers that kind of strength to the sensational feats of a professional lifter. For my part, I think the public is quite right. A man who can put a 400-lb. trunk on one shoulder and carry it up three flights of stairs without getting winded, has more bodily strength than the man who can "push up" a 100-lb. dumbbell, but who is unable to lift or carry really heavy objects. Most of these professional "Strong Men" could make the average baggage-smasher look like a child when it came to carrying trunks; but there are a great many amateurs who are so infatuated with biceps development that they never take the trouble to acquire the bodily strength of even the average day laborer.

Sometimes when you are out driving in your car you will see an automobile which has slewed sideways so that the rear wheels have gone down into a very deep and muddy gutter; and there may be three or four men grouped around it, trying to push it up on the road. Suppose, while you were watching, some well set-up young man would wave the four other men aside, brace his feet against the curb, put his shoulders against the back of the car and, with one motion, lift it out of the gutter. I saw this very thing done by a friend of mine, and what he actually did was just a simple leg lift; and as he could easily raise 2000 lbs. in a hip lift, it wasn't very much work for him to push the car out of the gutter. One of the young fellows, who had been riding in the car, said, "Gosh, that man must be stronger than all four of us put together!" He possibly was stronger than any two of them, but the reason that he, alone, was able to do more work than the crowd of them, was as much because he knew how to deliver his strength as because of the superior size and strength of his back and leg muscles. That is the one great virtue of training with weights: it teaches you to use your muscles in concert with one another. You should never depend on the strength of one set of muscles when it is possible to employ the strength of many muscles combined.

Any kind of exercise is good in its way; but there are only a few kinds of exercise which will create super-strength for you, or give you the build and appearance of a super-athlete. A great fault with most systems of light exercise is that they aim to develop the muscles individually. The directions say that "this exercise is for one part of the arms"; that the next is for another part of the arms, and so on through the whole body. It is possible, by performing light exercise (and repeating each exercise a great many times), to get a fairly nice development and fairly good-sized muscles; but the trouble is that after you have gotten the muscles, they are not very much good to you, because they have never been taught to act together. If all a man wants is moderate development and "just enough exercise to keep himself in condition," he can do more in that line by playing tennis in summer and handball in wintertime, than by doing free-hand movements or calisthenics; because tennis and handball do employ practically every muscle in the body and they do teach co- ordination.

In order to bring the legs to their full strength it is necessary to practice the variations of the full-squat with moderate weights, as well as practicing the "hand-and-thigh" and "Jefferson" exercises with fairly heavy weights. When you do a full squat you develop the muscles in the lower part of the thigh above the knee and, to a certain extent, you develop the inside and outside of the thighs; but, as the amount of weight you could use in the full squat is limited, you cannot, by that exercise, develop the upper part of the thighs to the limit. The thighs should be biggest right at the line of the crotch and they should taper to the knee. Arthur Saxon (who, in addition to being a wonderful lifter himself, was a great judge of lifters) said that when giving a new man the "once-over," he always looked to see whether the muscles in the lower part of the thigh were well developed; and that he considered it more necessary to have a fine development there than in the upper part of the thigh. While I agree with most of Mr. Saxon's ideas, I cannot subscribe to this one. I have seen many aspiring lifters who had odd-looking legs, because most of their leg work was aimed to develop these lower thigh muscles; and

42

my experience is that such men never have the driving force which is possessed by a man with powerful hips and big upper thighs. To get real super-strength you must work on the rule that your hips and thighs are as important to you as the hind legs are to a race horse. The horse, when running at full speed, gets almost all his driving power from the hind legs. The extended front legs catch his weight and then bring his body forward so that the hind legs can get in another thrust. When we come down to some of the bar-bell lifts, I will show you how the bell can be lifted to arms' length overhead, in a manner where the legs and back do so much of the work that the arms hardly seem to be doing more work than the race horse's front legs do in driving him along.

After you have mastered the other varieties of the leg exercises, you must practice the full squat, while holding a bell at arms' length above the head. The easiest way is to hold the bell aloft in one hand. Start with a 25-lb. bar-bell or dumbbell; push it to arms' length with the right hand, and keep the right arm stiff and straight, and then squat, as in Fig. 28. You will find it easier to keep your balance if you hold the left arm out to the side. The great virtue of this variation is that it absolutely compels you to keep the spine straight and do the bending with the legs. After you can do it easily with the bell supported in either the right or the left hand, try it with the bell held aloft in two hands, as in Fig. 29. Gradually increase the weight of the bell until you are able to squat easily and rapidly while holding aloft at least 75 lbs. Otto Arco, who was one of the few lifters who could raise double his own weight to arm's length above the head, told me that he practiced this variation in preference to all other leg exercises. Anyone who intends to try real bar-bell lifting, especially the quick lifts (such as the "snatch" and the "jerk") should be very careful to master this exercise, since it is about the only one which would teach him the balance and give him the confidence which is necessary for the successful completion of what we call the "quick lifts."

CHAPTER V

HARNESS AND PLATFORM LIFTING

There are so few who ever get a chance to practice this branch of lifting that it seems hardly worthwhile to describe it. However, it may help you to master the whole subject of super-strength if you learn the principles of back lifting. First comes the ordinary "back" or "platform lift," where the athlete gets under the weight and lifts it on his flat back. There are few photographs available, but you may be able to get an idea by looking at Fig. 30. This shows the Canadian, Wilfred Cabana, performing a back-lift with 3652 lbs. It is customary to place the weights on a platform which is rested on two trestles (or wooden horses), and these trestles must be so high that in order to get under the platform the athlete need bend his legs only a trifle at the knees. The body is at right angles to the legs, and the hands are supported on a strong stool, or low wooden horse, the arms slightly bent. The athlete raises the weight by simultaneously straightening the arms and the legs; but most of the work is done by the legs and, therefore, platform lifting is really more of a leg lift or a "hip-lift," than it is a true back lift. So far as I know the record in the back lift is held by the late Louis Cyr, who managed to raise about 4125 lbs. There are several other lifters who have raised in the neighborhood of 4000 lbs. Most men who use adjustable bar-bells for the purpose of developing their legs and back are able to make good records in the back-lift. In writing about the present crop of barbell lifters in Canada, Mr. Geo. Jowett says that DeCarie can do 3640 lbs. in the back lift; Cabana has done 3652, and that an amateur, by the name of La

Vallee, did 4000 lbs. on the first attempt. Another man, named La Tour, did 3214 lbs., and little Marineau, who weighs only 142 lbs., has raised 2809 lbs. on his back. Every one of the men just mentioned is a bar-bell lifter as well as a "back-lifter." In Canada, lifting clubs are equipped with the proper apparatus for "back" and "harness" lifting; whereas in this country it is hard to find a club which has a "back- lifting" platform.

I understand that in "back" and "harness" lifting, much more weight can be raised if the lifter is familiar with the correct positions, and the correct method of applying his strength. I have been told that in both these styles there is a method called the "wedge motion," in which the lifter shifts the weight a bit forward as he raises it, and that it is possible to lift more weight in this style than if you attempt to lift it directly upward. All that is fairly in the game. Naturally, if you wish to make your own individual record in any style of lift the thing that counts is the number of pounds you manage to raise; and it is perfectly proper to employ the method which has proven to be the best. People judge a man of super-strength by what he can do; not by what he might do if he knew how. Therefore, a man of great strength who knows how to employ that strength and raises 4000 lbs. on his back is a better athlete than the man of even greater strength who fails to lift 3600 lbs. because he does not know how to use his body.

Perhaps the best authority on this style of lifting is Mr. Warren Lincoln Travis, who, I believe, is the present world's champion. He specializes on this style of lifting, and long-continued practice has given him back and legs of enormous strength. One time I paid him a visit, and, after doing several other stunts, he showed me an endurance "hip-lift." He stood on a high platform, under which there was a 900-lb. weight. This weight was attached by a chain to a big belt, which was fastened around his hips. This lift is just about the same as the one shown in Fig. 21, except that the shape of the weight was different. At the start of the lift he stood upright, with his legs very slightly bent. Every time he would straighten his legs he would raise the weight about an inch; and, if my memory is right, he raised it about one hundred times in one minute. Although the gymnasium had a cement floor the whole building soon got to quivering as though an immense engine were running. As a matter of fact, the 900 lbs. was not a "lift" for Travis, but merely a developing exercise. Any feat that you can repeat many times is an exercise—not a lift.

Travis is an exception to the usual rule. Back lifting is his hobby, and bar-bell lifting just his occasional pastime; whereas most men of super-strength specialize on bar-bell lifting and only occasionally do "back" and "harness lifts"; but then, Travis has all the necessary paraphernalia which most of the other lifters lack. (While Mr. Travis is naturally proud of his records in back- lifting, he is prone to speak very disparagingly of his own ability as a bar-bell lifter. But that is just his way; he is a first-class barbell lifter and a darn sight better than he claims to be.)

In making a harness-lift, the athlete stands on a platform above the weight. The lower platform, which bears the weight, is usually suspended by four chains, which join to one chain which passes through a hole in the upper platform. This chain, in turn, is attached to the lifter's harness. In many cases, this harness consists of nothing more or less than a loop of broad leather strap, which passes from the lifter's shoulders and runs down to a point just in front of the hips. The athlete stands with his legs bent slightly at the knees, his body inclined forward from the hips, hands resting on a pair of railings or other firm supports, as in Fig. 3. In making the lift the athlete simultaneously straightens his legs and arms, and brings the trunk of his body to a vertical position. When only the shoulder strap is used the contents of the body are compressed, especially if the lifter arches his back

46

instead of keeping his spine straight. Real experts in harness-lifting use a belt around the hips as well as one around the shoulders, as this distributes the weight and enables them to lift far more than with only a shoulder belt. One can make a back- lifting platform without much trouble and at small expense; but a harness- lifting platform is an expensive affair, and, consequently, you rarely see "harness- lifting," except on the vaudeville stage. While it is a simple matter to estimate the amount of weight an athlete is raising in a back lift, it is a difficult thing to even guess the amount of weight a man is lifting with a harness. There are ways of rigging the lower platform which greatly reduce the amount of effort necessary to lift that platform. Fig. 31 is reproduced from Prof. Des Bonnet's book. It is shows a well-known, old-time lifter at the completion of a harness-lift; but Des Bonnet says that when the lifter did this stunt as an exhibition feat he had the platform so rigged that he actually lifted only one-tenth of the weight; that is when he had 2400 lbs. on the lower platform he could raise it with no more exertion than if he had a 240-lb. weight attached by a single chain to his neck harness. However, this is not a discussion of the methods of professional performers, and there are comparatively few of these professionals who resort to trickery in order to make their strength seem more surprising. Most of them are so very strong that they do not have to use any artificial aids to enable them to juggle with, or lift enormous weights.

One famous "Strong Man" told me that in harness-lifting it was a great mistake to stand in the position shown in Fig. 3, and that one should never rest the hands on the side supports. He said that the lifter should stand with the left foot slightly in advance of the right foot, and that the side supports should be so high that he could rest his elbows on them. Then, when he was ready to lift the weight, he should thrust forward as well as upward, which seems to be the same "wedge motion" that the experts use in back-lifting.

47

"Harness-lifting" is no game for the weak or untrained man, and for that matter, neither is back-lifting. If, however, a man developed the back and legs by practicing the back and leg exercises, in Chapters II and IV he can safely practice harness-lifting or back-lifting. In a book which I wrote a dozen years ago I said that the average 170-lb. amateur, who could lift a 250-lb. bar-bell above his head (with both hands), should be able to do 2500 or 3000 lbs. in a "back" or "harness-lift"; and I am still of that opinion.

The fact that you may never have a chance to try a back-lift or a harness-lift does not mean that you should fail to practice the back and leg exercises with weights running from 50 to 500 lbs., according to the exercise. Five hundred pounds sounds like a whole lot; but since there are lots of porters, stevedores and day laborers who move or lift 500-lb. cases and crates all morning and all afternoon, then any man scientifically trained can use those weights for a few minutes with perfect safety.

This reminds me that I am frequently asked that, if handling heavy weights creates great strength, why it is that some of these porters do not develop enormous strength. Some of them do, although the majority of them do not. You would think that a foundry man who spends all his day in carrying heavy ladles of molten metal, or in lifting heavy castings would become enormously strong, and that muscles would stick out all over him. Likewise, you'd think that a coal heaver would naturally develop a back of prodigious strength. The reason why such men do not develop is because they have too much of such work, and that they have to continue working for hours after the body has become tired from the exertion in the first part of the morning. That, by the way, is one reason why heavy laborers sometimes appear to be loafing on the job. The truth is, their work is so exacting that if they worked at full tilt they would be "all in" by 10 A.M. They are compelled to economize their strength and to work at a slow, steady gait, if they are going to last out the eight-hour day. The coal shoveler or ditch digger must have frequent rests. Their work is neither light enough to be easy nor heavy enough to force them to use great muscular strength. Frequently their diet is almost suicidal, and their hours of sleep insufficient. Any man who uses weights scientifically three or four hours a week can become vastly stronger and infinitely better developed than the average man who earns his bread by heavy labor.

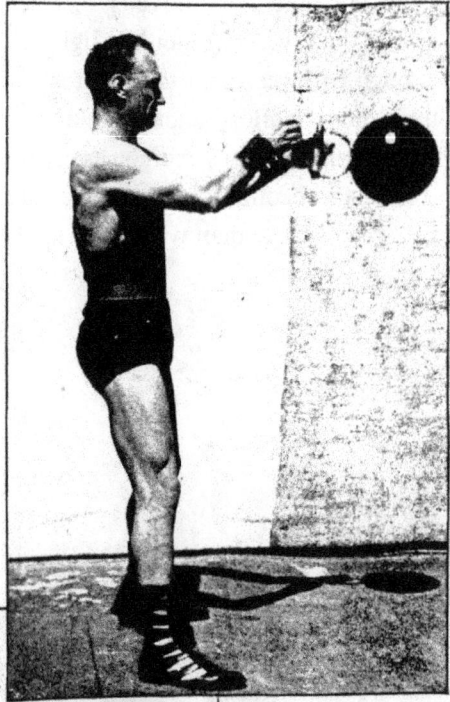

Fig. 13

Plate 7, Figures 12 and 13. One of the best exercises for teaching the leg and back muscles to act in concert. The most important feature of this exercise is that it teaches you to lift with a flat back. Note that in Fig. 12 the athlete has leaned over by bending the legs a trifle at the knees, and inclining the body forward at the hips, and that the spine is kept absolutely straight

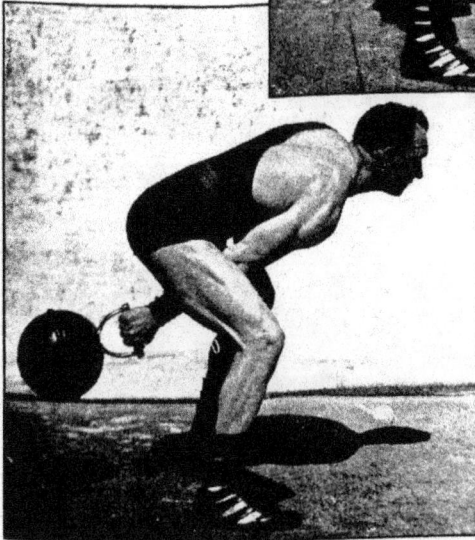

Fig. 12

Although the left hand cannot be seen in Fig. 12, it is resting on the left knee. When the swing is made with the left hand, the right hand must rest on the right knee

50

PLATE 8

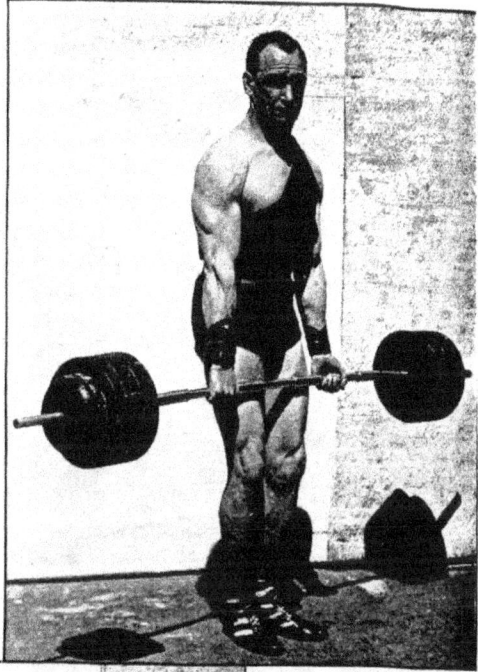

Fig. 15

Plate 8, Figures 14 and 15. These two illustrations show the official method of performing the "Deadweight Lift." The athlete should stand with heels together, and then lean over, by arching the back and b e n d i n g the legs slightly at the knees. The bar-bell is grasped in the manner shown with the palms of the hands pointing in opposite directions

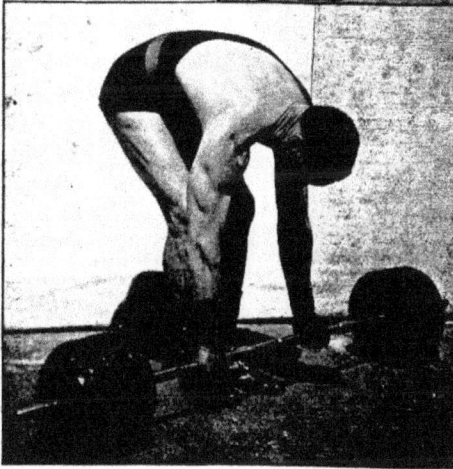

Fig. 14

The weight is then lifted directly up until the athlete stands erect, as in Fig. 15 (above). In posing for these pictures, Mr. Donald used only 330 lbs. of weight, which is more than 100 lbs. less than he could do in this style

PLATE 9

Fig. 16

Plate 9, Figure 17 (below), shows the method of performing the "Hand and Thigh" lift on a platform. Figure 16 (above), shows how you can practice this lift with a bar-bell by utilizing a pair of ropes, and the dumbbell handle from your outfit

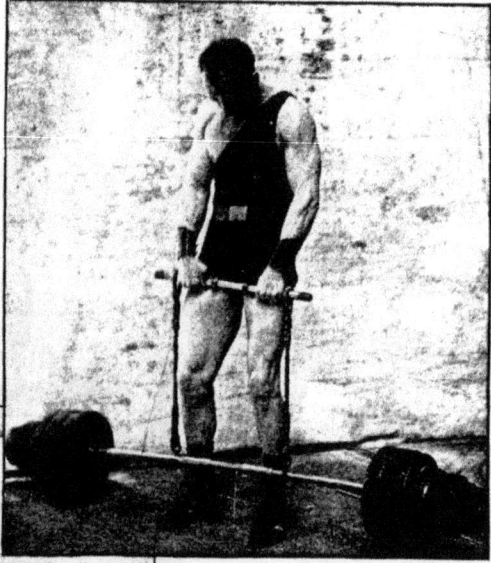

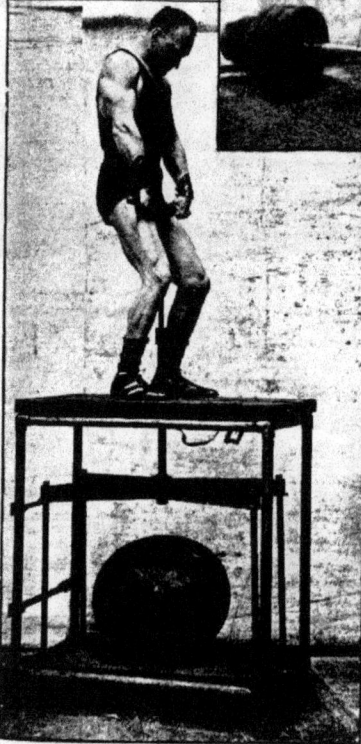

Fig. 17

Mr. Donald, being unfamiliar with this lift, placed his hands a bit too low. The knuckles should have rested right in the bend of the leg. Nevertheless, he lifted 500 lbs. in the platform with the utmost ease, and when using a 400-lb. bar-bell, he lifted it several times in succession. With a few days' practice at the correct style, he could easily do 1,200 lbs. This is far the easiest method to lift a heavy weight from the ground

PLATE 10

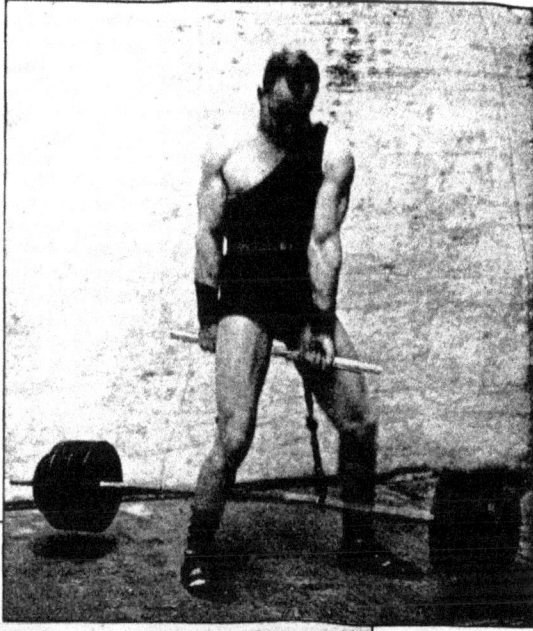

Fig. 18

Plate 10, Figure 18 (a b o v e), shows how you can practice the "Jefferson" lift with a bar-bell, a pair of ropes, and the dumb-bell h a n d l e. Owing to the s t r a i n of the grip, it is not possible to lift as much in this way as by the "H a n d a n d Thigh" method.

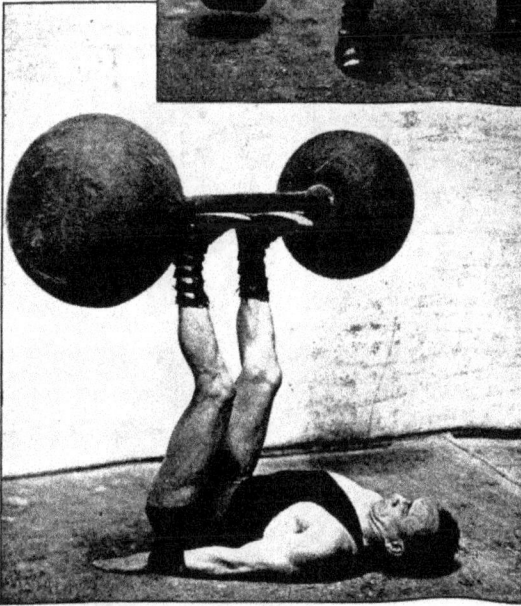

Fig. 19

F i g u r e 19 (be-low), illustrates the method of lift-i n g a h e a v y w e i g h t on the soles of the feet. T h e f a m o u s A r t h u r Saxon lifted over 2,000 lbs. in this style. The bell used in this picture is a stage bell. It is not n e a r l y as heavy as it looks.

PLATE 11

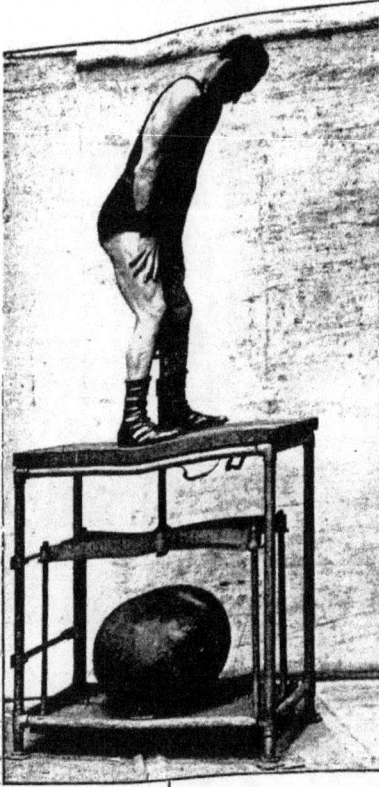

Fig. 20

Plate 11, Figure 20 (below), shows the "Leg" lift with a light bar-bell, performed as an exercise to develop the muscles on the back of the thighs

Fig. 21

Figure 21 (above), shows the "Hip" lift on a platform. The belt, which passes around the waist, can hardly be seen in this picture

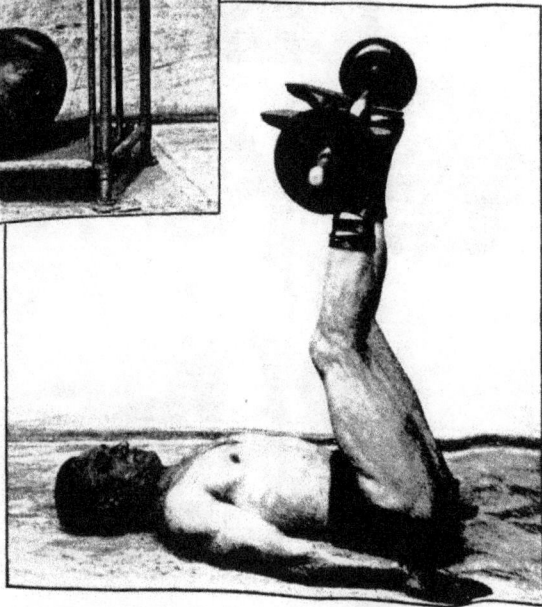

PLATE 12

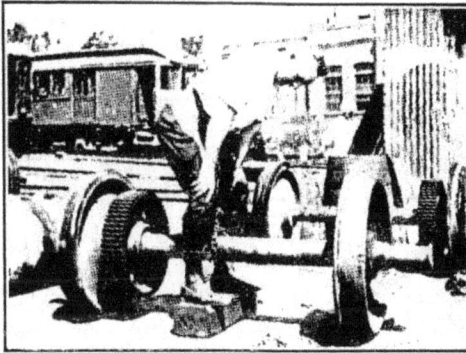

Fig. 22

Plate 12, Figure 22 (above), shows Roy Smith making a correct "Hip-lift" w i t h 2,250 lbs. The belt, which is made of w h i t e webbing, can easily be seen in this picture

Mr. Smith lifted this enormous weight one inch off the ground, a feat which calls for enormous strength in the legs. He developed that strength by practicing the modification of the "Jefferson" lift, shown in Figure 23 (below)

Fig. 23

In performing this exercise, the legs are bent no further than shown in the picture. Mr. Smith uses 400 lbs. in doing this exercise, which is more than most men can lift once that high f r o m t h e ground. This exercise is made easier if you practice it in the style shown in Figure 18

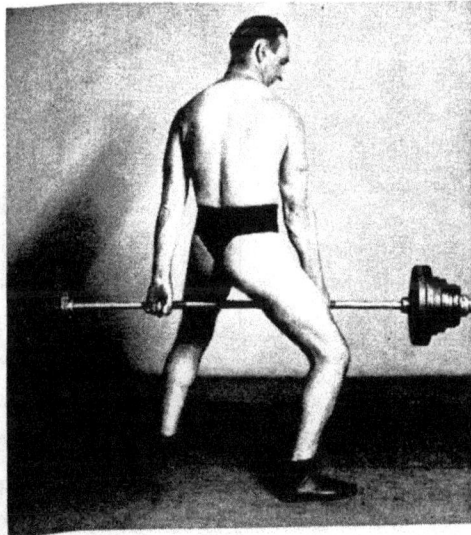

PLATE 13

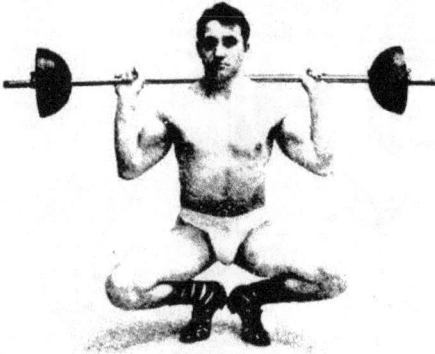

Fig. 25

Figure 25 (below). In this style the athlete stands with the feet close together, and parallel to each other, holds the dumbbell behind him, and as he squats, he forces the knees directly forward in order to develop the muscles on the inside of the thighs, right above the knee

Fig. 24

Plate 13, Figure 24 (above), shows the easiest method of doing the "Squat" or "Deep-knee-bend" to develop the muscles of the thighs. In this style, the athlete stands with the heels close together, and the toes turned outwards. As he squats, he forces the knees as far apart as possible in order to throw as much work as possible on the muscles of the outer sides of the thighs

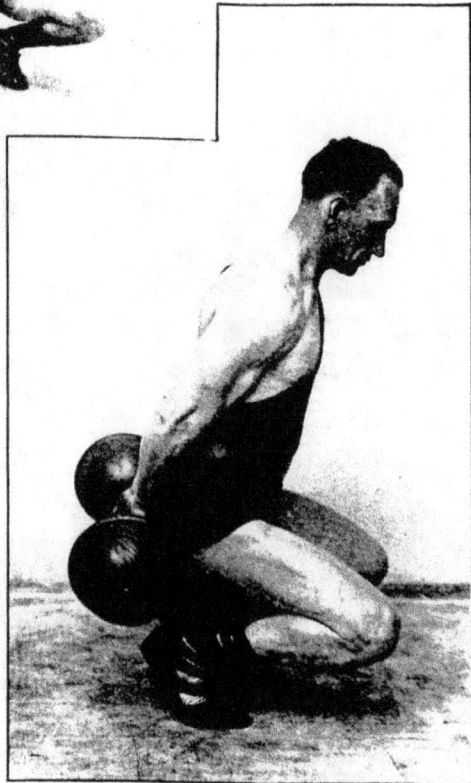

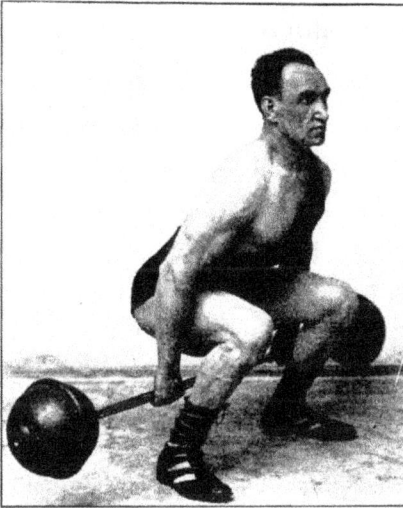

PLATE 14

Fig. 26

Plate 14, Figure 26 (above). A variation of the "Squat," which develops the muscles on the inside of the thighs. The feet should be 18 inches apart, the toes turned outward, and the heels are not allowed to leave the ground

Fig. 27

Figure 27 (below) shows Henry Steinborn half-way down in the "Squat". This man can squat two or three times in succession with 500 lbs. across the shoulders. At the completion of the squat, he goes even further down than Donald does in Figure 26

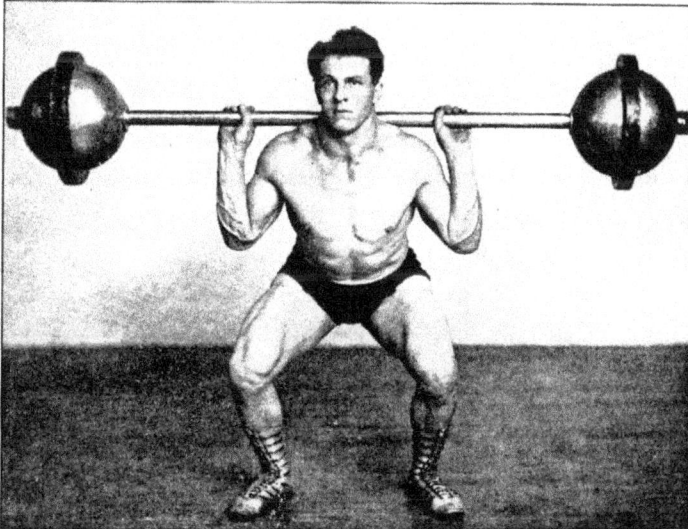

CHAPTER VI

THE SIDES

In his book on physical education, Dr. Felix Oswald said, in some parts of England, the title of "the strongest man in the neighborhood" was awarded to the man who could take the heaviest weight on his shoulder and walk with it the longest distance with the firmest step. That, by the way, is a very fair test of bodily strength. If a man is weak in the back he cannot even get the weight on his shoulder in the first place. If he is weak in the knees (that is, if his leg muscles are weak) his legs will "buckle" at the knees, and he will shamble along after he has carried the weight a very short distance; and a little after that he will collapse entirely under the weight. A man with strong back and legs might successfully carry a weight which rested on both shoulders; but, unless he had strong sides he wouldn't get very far with the weight on one shoulder, because when you do have a heavy weight on one shoulder the tendency of the weight is to pull you over sideways. With even a moderately heavy weight on the right shoulder the tendency is to thrust the hips toward the right in order to better balance the weight. When the hips are thus thrust out of their proper alignment, it becomes impossible to walk with a firm, even tread. Again, no man can hold a heavy weight on the shoulder unless he has great strength in the trapezius muscle, which lifts, or sustains the shoulder. If the trapezius is weak, the shoulder under the weight will slump, and the weight will roll off. There is a concrete example of what I mean by bodily strength; and I again want to emphasize the fact that super- strength is immense bodily strength, and not just arm-strength. If you have ever tried to carry a 200-lb. box or trunk on the shoulder, it will make you appreciate the bodily strength of a man like Horace Barre, who once put a 1270-lb. bar-bell on one shoulder and walked about fifty feet with it.

If you examine the statues of the ancient Greek athletes and demigods, you will find that there is very little delineation of the muscles. There are no bunches of muscles on the arms or legs; and about the only muscles which are plainly outlined are the pectoral muscles on the breast and the muscles at the sides of the waist. In modern men, you find the side-muscles finely developed only in wrestlers, in bar-bell lifters and in laborers whose daily work requires them to carry heavy weights in one hand, or upon one shoulder. Some gymnasts and light-exercise enthusiasts get a partial development of the side-muscles, and if they bend sideways, they can make the side-muscles apparent; whereas, if a man has trained with bar-bells, his side-muscles are at all times as apparent as the muscles on his chest or shoulders.

One of the easiest ways to develop the side-muscles is to take a very heavy weight in one hand and walk around the room. If the weight is in the right hand, it tends to pull you over to the right; and therefore, the muscle on the left side of the waist is very busy in its efforts to hold the trunk upright. The main trouble with this exercise is that your fingers will give out before your side-muscles do. Another simple exercise is to take a 40- or 50-lb. dumbbell in one hand, to keep the legs upright and bend over sideways at the waist, as in Fig. 32. You should bend over and straighten up again, several times in succession. In Fig. 32, the muscle at the right side of the waist is plainly visible, but it is the muscle on the left which is doing the work, as it is that muscle which straightens the body after you bend it over. Another exercise for the side is to hold a bar-bell across the shoulders, to stand with the feet far apart and firmly braced; then bend the body first to the right and then to the left. The objection to that style is that it never allows you to get a full contraction of the muscles on either side.

The very best exercise for developing the sides is the one illustrated in Fig. 33. You start out by taking a 25-lb. dumbbell and pushing it to arm's length with the right hand; then you step forward with the left foot, so that the heel of that foot is about 20 inches away from the inside of the right foot, the toes being turned slightly outwards. Keep the right leg straight; bend the left leg at the knee; then, still holding the bell aloft, lean over and touch the left toes with the finger-tips of the left hand. Straighten up again and repeat several times without lowering the bell. It is very much easier to do this exercise if, when you have the bell in your right hand, you rest most of the weight on the advanced left foot, as this makes it easier to bend the body over. When you first try this exercise you will find it difficult, because the hand holding the dumbbell will sway around in a manner which will make you think you're going to lose your balance; and so you will, unless you keep your gaze fastened on the dumbbell. Never make the mistake of looking down to see where your left foot is, because your hand will find the foot automatically. Keep watching the bell and you will have no trouble in keeping your balance. The arm which holds the bell, should be perpendicular to the floor at all times. As you stand up, both legs should be straight for an instant; and then you can bend the left knee and rest your weight on the left foot as you bend over. (Of course, all these directions are exactly reversed when you have the bell in the left hand.) In performing any kind of work, lift or exercise, the body is rarely bent directly to the side. Almost always the bend is sideways— and partly to the front. The virtue of this exercise is that it teaches your side-muscles to work in harmony with the lower-back muscles, and that it helps to develop the muscles which rotate the trunk on its own axis. Furthermore, it is simply invaluable training if you wish to learn, later on, to lift heavy weights above the head by the method known as the "bent press."

In my talk about back-strength, I compared the hips to the

centre of a hinge, and said that there must be equal strength in both sides of the hinge. This is equally true, no matter of which joint you are speaking. It is impossible to exercise the side muscles by themselves any more than you can use the back muscles by themselves. When you bend the body sideways, you call into vigorous action not only the muscles at the side of the waist, but the muscles on the outside of the thighs. Therefore, any athlete with strikingly developed muscles at the side of the waist is practically bound to have an equally striking development on the outside of the thighs. Turn over the pages of this book and look at the pictures of Sandow, Saxon, Matysek, Nordquest, Carr, or any of the other men who have made great records in the one-arm bent press, and you will see that the thighs of all these men have a great, sweeping curve on the outer side of the leg, from the knee to the hip-bone. Following the same principle, any man with highly developed muscles along the spine is almost sure to have swelling biceps muscles on the back of the thigh, and calves of the legs which are deep from front to back. Likewise, any athlete with fine abdominal muscles will have fine muscles on the front of the thigh, I will modify that last statement. It is possible to develop the abdominal muscles in a certain way without bringing out much development on the front of the thigh. In my opinion, that is a foolish way to develop any set of muscles. Muscles are not just for appearance, but for use; and if your front-thighs and abdominal muscles are exercised in concert, they will be much better developed and very much stronger than if you attempt to develop the abdominal muscles alone. Occasionally you see a man who, by the so-called "muscle-spinning" process, has acquired quite fine development of many individual muscles; but it is very rarely that such men have anything more than the average strength. Their muscles have been developed through first placing the body in a position which allows a particular muscle to get in the position of extreme contraction, and then

61

contracting and releasing it just by an effort of the will. Muscles developed in this way have some size and some shape, but practically no power and absolutely no co-ordination. The Germans used to have a complicated word describing this condition. When translated, it meant "A-man-who-is-like-a- shop - keeper-who -has-all-his-goods-in-the-window-and-nothing-on-the-shelves-in-his-store." There is a great difference in the quality of a muscle which has been developed by work; that is, by contracting against actual resistance, and a muscle which has been developed simply by continued contractions against no resistance. I have taught many a man how to get a fair arm-development by putting his arm in two different positions and flexing first the biceps and then the triceps muscle by an effort of the will; but I always warn such men that muscles developed in this way are apt to be "puffy" and not capable of doing any real work.

The muscles at the sides of the waist are often overlooked by devotees of light-exercise, who prefer to devote their time to developing the showy muscles on the arms and shoulders. It is possible to get a fine arm and shoulder development without any real hard work; because most arm exercises are not vigorous enough to cause fatigue. (That is why the teacher who advertises that he has some "easy and pleasant method" of becoming strong, almost always makes you specialize on arm-exercises.) Furthermore, it explains why so many men who have spent years in cultivating their arms muscles, have never acquired the bodily strength and development which raises a man into the class of the super-strong. Whatever you do, don't fall into the error of neglecting the exercises for the legs, back and sides. When you come to the description of some of the overhead bar-bell lifts, you will find that instead of these lifts being performed solely by the strength of the arms, the bulk of the work is done by the back, leg and side muscles you have developed by doing the exercises in the preceding chapters.

CHAPTER VII

THE ABDOMINAL MUSCLES

At the present time the development of the abdominal muscles has become almost a fad with some physical culturists. If you pick up a magazine devoted to exercises you are almost sure to find some pictures showing young men with their bodies bent forward so as to make the muscles on the front of the abdomen stand out in ridges.

Since the muscles along the front of the abdomen are fastened at top to the breast-bone, and at the bottom to the bones of the pelvis, it follows that contraction of these muscles bends the body forward and brings the chest closer to the knees.

I can see the importance of these abdominal muscles, but I think that no man should cultivate them and leave his back-muscles neglected. Eugen Sandow, who "started" so many other things, is responsible for the craze for abdominal development. The muscles on the front of his abdomen were phenomenal; but not a bit more phenomenal than the muscles on his back. Up to the time that he made his debut as a vaudeville performer, it was customary for a professional "Strong Man" to work in a high-necked jersey; and as these men never stripped or did muscle-poses in a lighted cabinet, the people who saw their acts never got a chance to see the remarkable development of the abdominal muscles which many of them possessed.

In a real "Strong Man" the muscles on the front of the abdomen should be plainly visible when the body is held erect. It should not be necessary to bend the body over, as in Fig. 34, in order to make these muscles noticeable. If you look at the picture of Sandow in Fig. 35, you can trace the outline of the abdominal muscles; even though in this pose, he is actually leaning slightly backwards. In his case, these muscles were so noticeable that out of a hundred people who saw him pose, ninety-nine would remember the development of his abdominal muscles, where only one would notice the wonderful cables of muscle along either side of his spine.

As a rule, I can say that most men and boys who take up bodybuilding exercise end up by having a better development on the front of their bodies than on the back of their bodies. This is due to their constant habit of standing in front of a mirror and studying their own development. It is easy for them to see the outline of the muscles on the chest, those on the front of the abdomen and the muscles on the front of the thighs.

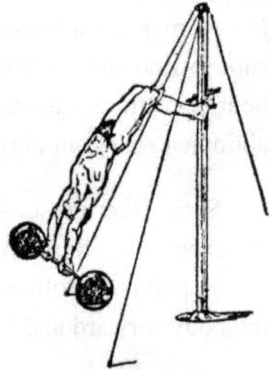

Fig. 37

They see the width of the calves of the legs, and if it seems insufficient, they will do exercises to make the calves wider, forgetting that the important thing is to make the calves deep from front to back. Similarly, they will work hard to make the thighs look wider and never once think of the vitally important muscles on the back of the thigh, which they never see in the mirror. Worst of all, they do far more exercises for the muscles on the breast and on the front of the abdomen, than for the muscles on the back of the body.

I am not trying to discourage the developing of the abdominal muscles, but to make you realize their place and proportion in your whole muscular get-up. Anyone who has practiced even the simplest kinds of exercise is familiar with the two usual exercises which develop the abdominal muscles. In both exercises you lie flat on the back. In one of them you raise the legs to a perpendicular position; and in the other you keep the legs on the floor by placing a weight across the ankles, and then you bring the body to a perpendicular position. The first

64

exercise, where you raise the legs, seems to develop the lower part of the abdominal muscles; that is, the part in the neighborhood of the groin. In the other exercise, where you raise the body, most of the work is done by the upper fibers, where they attach to the breast-bone. (If a fat man carries most of the surplus flesh around the hips, he should practice raising the legs; but if most of the surplus is on the upper part of the abdomen, he should practice the other variation.) But these two exercises are merely "kindergarten stuff," and they have no place in the training-schedule of the super-strong. They are so easy that men have been known to bring the body to the perpendicular position 2000 times in succession; and almost anyone can, in a few weeks' practice, learn to repeat either movement from 25 to 50 times. Anyone who can do that much, can safely start doing the body- raising movement while holding a weight at the back of the neck, as in Fig. 36. The beginner can start with 10 or 15 lbs., and he will find that he can increase quite rapidly, and that it soon becomes no more trouble to do the exercise with 50 lbs. than it formerly was with 15 lbs. When he gets this far along, he should adopt a more strenuous method. (In some of our cities no candidate is accepted for the police-force unless he can do this exercise with 40 lbs.).

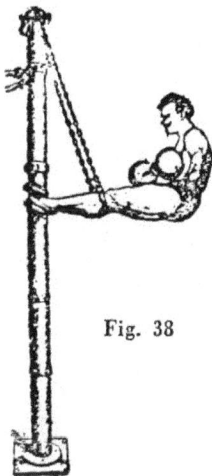
Fig. 38

The next step in abdominal development is to sit on a bench or a chair and then lean back and pick up a light bar-bell, rest it on the upper-chest, and bring the body to a sitting position. Naturally, the feet have to be fastened to the floor, and the customary thing is to either put the toes under a strap or else to put the insteps under a heavy bar-bell. This variation should not be attempted until it is easy to use 50 lbs. in the preceding

65

method, and then you should start on the chair with 10 or 15 lbs. When you can make several repetitions with 50 lbs., it is time for you to graduate into Roman-chair or Roman-column work.

Now we are coming to really advanced abdominal exercises. In all the previous variations, where you rest the body, your weight has been supported at the hips and all the bending has been done from the hip-joint. In the Roman-chair and Roman-column work, the support is at the knees, which makes it much more difficult; because, for one thing, the leverage is longer, and for another thing, the work is shared between the abdominal muscles and the muscles of the hips and thighs. Of the two kinds of apparatus, the column is much preferable. If you refer to Fig. 37, you will see that there are rests for the feet, and that most of the athlete's weight is carried by the chains fastened at one end of the post, and at the other end to straps buckled around the upper part of the calves. In a properly arranged Roman-column, when the athlete leans back and throws his weight against the chains, the knee-joint should be but little higher than the ankle-joint. The first exercise in the Roman-column is to learn to get in the sitting position shown in Fig. 38, which, by the way, is much harder than you would think. Then you learn to bend backwards and lower the body until the finger-tips touch the floor, as in Fig. 39. The real work comes in raising the body again to the sitting position, and no one should even attempt the stunt unless the muscles of the abdomen and groin have been developed and strengthened by the preceding exercises. Since, on your first attempt to use a column, you might find it impossible to bring your body up, you should always have a friend present to rescue you, if necessary, from the head-downward position. During the first week's practice you will gain

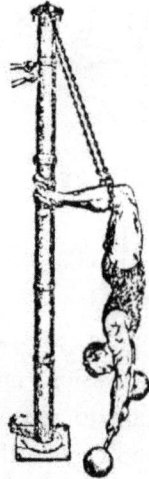

Fig. 39

66

in strength at a surprising rate; and while the first day you may not be able to bring your body up even once, on the seventh day you will do it many times with the utmost ease. Then is time to start with a light bar-bell; ten or fifteen pounds is enough to begin with. You have to lift it from the floor, hold it against the bend of the hips, and then bring it with you to the sitting position. You can make the work harder either by increasing the weight of the bell or by holding it close to the chin instead of in front of the hips. The further the weight is away from the knees, the more strength it takes to raise the bell and the body. After a month's practice you will suddenly awake to the fact that you have a degree of bodily strength which is entirely new and most pleasing; and you will wonder why it was that you wasted so many weary months trying to get real strength by performing the kindergarten exercises which started this chapter.

Since few Roman-columns are available, many athletes have to resort to the use of the Roman-chair, which is illustrated in Fig. 40. Such chairs have to be of very strong construction. The straps on the seat of the chair hold the athlete's feet firmly in place, and the top of the chair is padded. The back and seat should be inclined as in Fig. 40, and not upright and horizontal as in the ordinary chair. My objection to the chair is that you have to bend the body back farther in order to reach the ground. In the pictures of the Roman- column, you will see that when the body is down it is at right angles to the calves of the legs; and in the pictures of the Roman-chair, the body has to be bent beyond the right angle.

Undoubtedly the idea of the Roman-column occurred to some gymnast or athlete who was familiar with the parallel-bars. It is possible to do Roman-column work on a pair of parallels, providing the bars are not too far apart. All you have to do is to sit sideways, with the insteps under one bar and the bend of your knees over the other bar. Since most parallel-bars are adjustable, both in height and in width, you can fix them so that your legs will stretch across the open space between the bars, and so that when you are hanging head-downwards, your finger-tips just sweep the floor. It is easier to do the work on a Roman-column, because the leg-straps and the foot-rests are padded; but if you can't find a Roman- column or chair, there is nothing to prevent your trying the column exercises on a pair of parallels.

I'm afraid that some of you will be discouraged when you read this chapter, and that you will decide to give up all idea of getting to be super-strong if it is necessary to do stunts like this. A man who has only average strength is hardly able to imagine what it feels like to be really strong. Let me assure you that a man who has gotten super-strength by practicing with weights thinks no more of getting on a Roman-column and doing an exercise three or four times with a 50-lb. bar-bell than you would think of lying flat on the back and raising your legs in the air three or four times in succession. I realize that if you have never tried it, Roman- column work seems at first glance to be a most difficult and dangerous form of exercise; just as the performance of a Kreisler or a Heifetz seems highly difficult and complicated to the man who has never taken a lesson in violin playing. You probably have thought that it would take the strength of a Hercules to do Roman-column work. That is more or less true; but the point is, that if you can learn to do it, you will get the strength of a Hercules; and once you have that strength and the corresponding muscular development, you will be surprised at how easily you can retain it, and how little work is necessary to keep the body at the highest pitch of condition. Make up your mind to this: If you ever get to be super-strong, you will thereafter have no patience with the "light" exercises which formerly seemed to be all-sufficient. If you can get on a Roman-column and repeat the exercise a few times in the course of one minute, why should you spend a half-hour lying on the floor and raising first the legs and then the body to the perpendicular position ? When you get so that you can handle 600 or 800 lbs. in a hand-and-thigh lift, and that five minutes' practice per week keeps your back and leg muscles in fine shape, you will have neither the time nor inclination to bend over and touch your toes 200 or 300 times in succession.

So far as I am aware, there are no records for Roman-column work, because it is not a competitive lift, but is used either as an exhibition stunt or as a developing exercise. When using it as an exercise, you should never push yourself to the limit of your strength, but should always keep a factor of reserve. It is not necessary to repeat the exercise every day, two or three times a week being sufficient to keep the muscles growing in size and strength. Fig. 40 is a sample of the bodily strength which can be created in this method. Few ordinary athletes can hold the body horizontally when the feet are strapped to a Roman-chair. This man can hold his own weight, plus the weight of a 100-lb. man at arms' length. If the other man were resting across the lifter's thighs, the stunt would be easy. In this instance it is hard, because the extra weight is right above the lifter's chest.

CHAPTER VIII

THE CHEST

In the minds of most of you the word "chest" means the front part of your upper-body; and when you say "chest muscles," what you really mean is the "pectorals" or muscles. Since the word "chest" means "box," your chest is your rib-box. When you take your chest-measurement, you pass the tape all around the body, and you will be disappointed, or pleased, according to the size of your rib-box. If the rib-box is small, you will never show a really big chest measurement, even if the muscles on the breast and upper back are thick and highly developed. On the other hand, the man who has a really big rib-box always shows a fine chest measurement, even if the upper-body muscles are comparatively under-developed. When the rib-box itself is large and the exterior muscles are highly developed, then you can get a phenomenal chest measurement, like that of Lange, Hackenschmidt and other devotees of bar-bell exercise.

The chest and lungs are the storehouses of your power. A big rib-box means plenty of room for the lungs. Big lungs are of immense value to the super-strong man. They enable him to keep up for many minutes at a time exertions which would exhaust the ordinary individual in the course of a few seconds.

Therefore, your first aim should be to increase the size of the rib-box; and even if you do not intend to try for super-strength, or if you are not interested in any other kind of exercise, I most earnestly recommend you to practise the movement described in the following paragraphs. A few months' daily practice will increase the girth of your rib-box by several inches. As the rib box grows larger, the shoulders will get proportionately broader; the lungs will get bigger; and you will find that you will have vastly more endurance as the size and power of the lungs increases. Furthermore, you will find that your arms and legs will develop almost automatically. A big-chested man can get arm and leg development at a much more rapid pace than can the man who has a small rib-box, and correspondingly small lungs. It is comparatively easy to "pack" muscle on the upper-back; and it is no trouble at all to get big muscles on the breast; but the man who has such development of the superficial muscles, while he may present a nice appearance, will not have super-strength. I have found that if a man can increase the girth of the rib-box by six or eight inches, that his shoulder blades will set themselves farther apart, thus widening his upper-back; also, that in some mysterious way the shoulders seem to re-adjust themselves in a way that makes for longer leverage, and hence greater power, in the muscles on the upper-body. You will often find that a broad-shouldered man with moderate development is much stronger than a heavy-muscled man who has narrow shoulders. This is due, in part, to the extra lung capacity; that is, the bigger "power-storehouse" which the broad-shouldered man possesses; and, in part, to muscular leverage. It is almost impossible to conceive a really big-chested man with narrow shoulders; just as it is impossible to make a mental picture of a man with, say a 45-inch chest, with shoulders only 16 or 17 inches in breadth. A man with a 32-inch chest will probably measure less than 16 inches from the point of one shoulder to the other; a man with a 40-inch chest will go about 19 inches across the shoulders; whereas, a giant like Zottman has shoulders nearly 24 inches across, to match his 46-inch chest.

Part of the width of the shoulders is due to the development of the deltoid muscles on the point of the shoulders; and in most big- chested men these muscles are very thick and strong. The deltoids are involved in any scheme for chest development; by which I mean that in order to increase the size of the true chest, it is necessary to perform exercises which involve the deltoid muscles.

PLATE 15

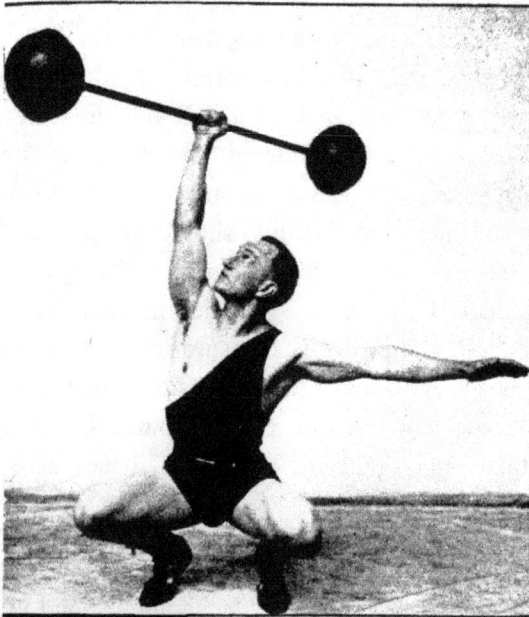

Fig. 28

Plate 15, Figure 28 (a b o v e), shows the full squat, with the bell held aloft in one hand. You s h o u l d l e a r n t h i s method before you attempt the style shown in Figure 29 (below), where the bell is held aloft with two hands. This style of squatting throws all the work on the legs, as it is n e c e s s a r y to keep the body upright, and the spine straight

Fig. 29

Continued practice of these exercises will give you the confidence, a n d teach you the balance necessary to successfully complete the quick lifts, such as the "Snatch" and the "Jerk"

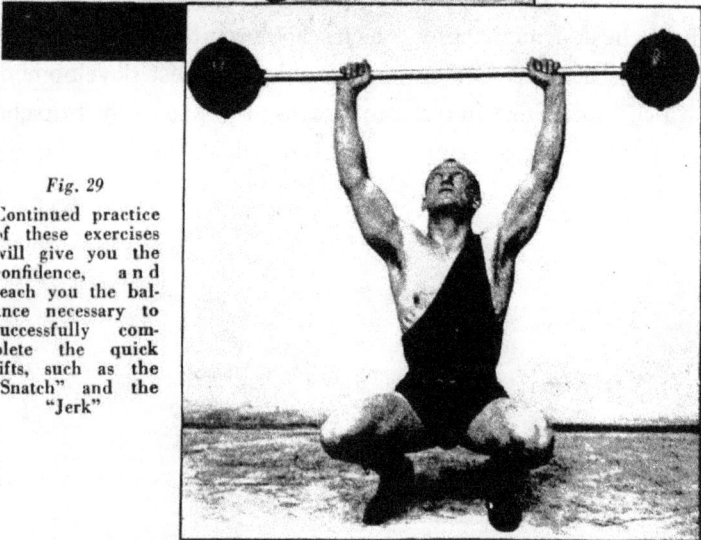

PLATE 16

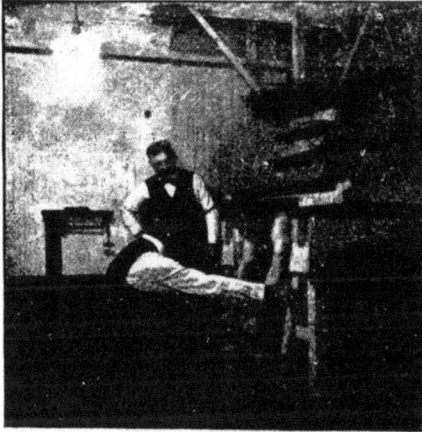

Fig. 30

Plate 16, Figure 30 (above) shows Wilford Cabana lift ing 3,652 lbs. on his back The record in the back lift is 4,125 lbs., made by the late Louis Cyr.

Fig. 31

Figure 31 (below), shows one of the old-time "Strong Men" doing a "Harness" lift. This picture is reproduced f r o m Prof. Des Bonnette's book, "The Kings of Strength." The Professor says that on this platform the supporting chains were so arranged that the work of lifting was much lightened

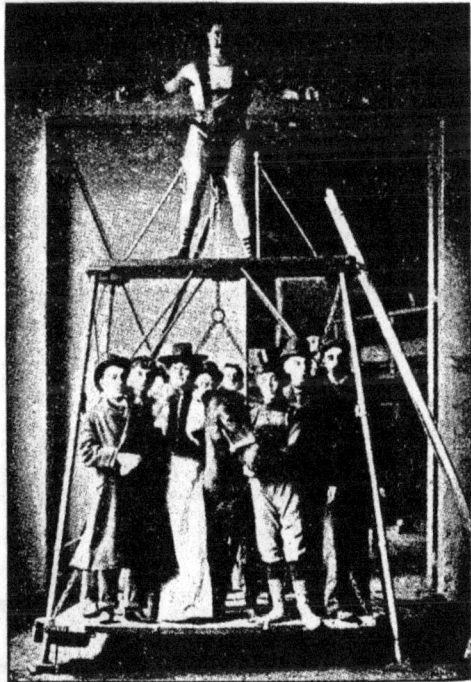

73

PLATE 17

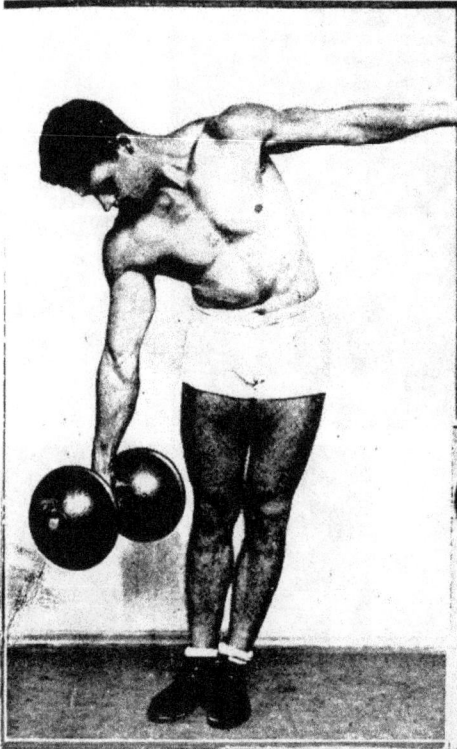

Fig. 32

Plate 17, F i g u r e 32 (above).   The easiest exercise to de- velop the mus- cles at the sides of the waist. The athlete stands with the legs close together, and does all the bending at the waist. In the picture the muscle on the right side of the waist shows up because it is com- pressed, but it is the muscle on the left side of the waist which will bring the body again to the vertical position

Fig. 33

Figure 33 (below). A more difficult exercise for the sides, and one which develops not only the side muscles, but also the muscles of the small of the back, and the under- side of the thighs. This movement is in- valuable training for those who wish to master the "Bent Press" lift

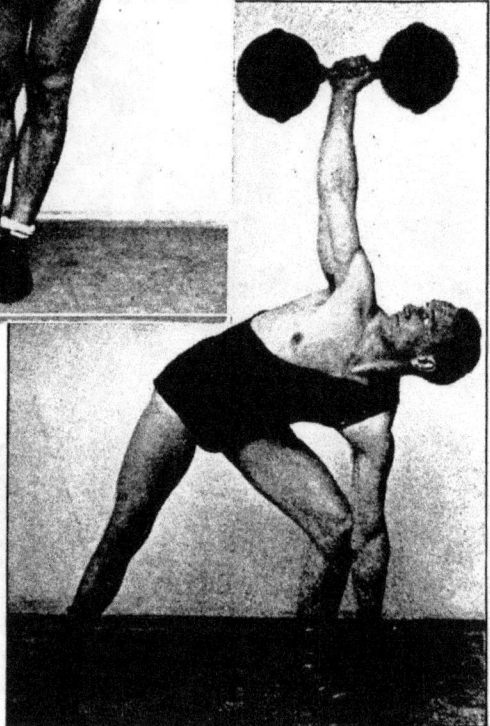

PLATE 18

Fig. 34

Plate 18, Figure 34 (above), is a pose of Albert Tauscher, in which he is leaning slightly forward in order to contract, and display his abdominal muscles

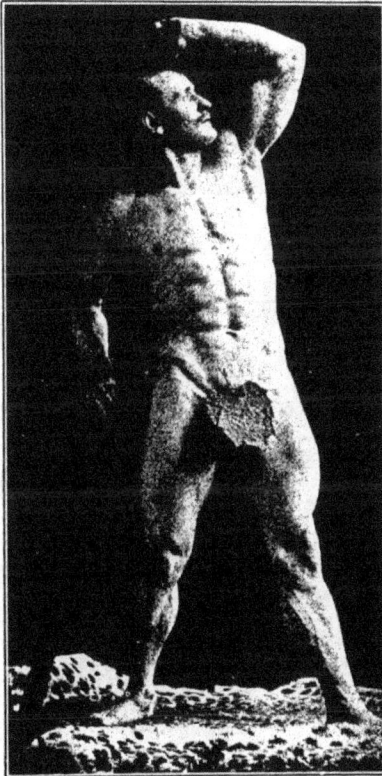

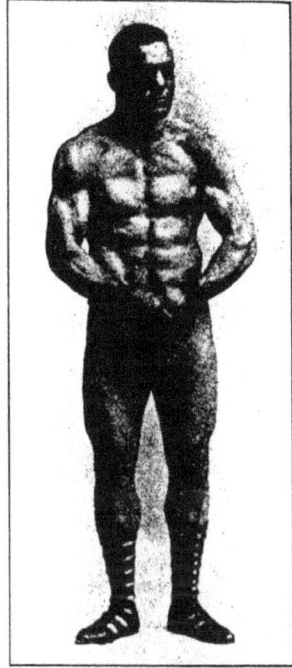

Fig. 35

Figure 35 (below), is an old photograph of Sandow, taken by Otto Sarony. Sandow's abdominal muscles were so highly developed that they were plainly evident even when he leaned slightly backwards, as in this pose

PLATE 19

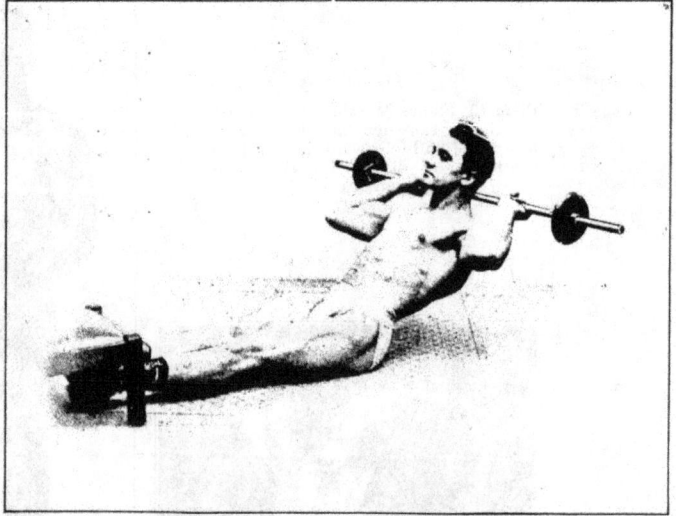

Fₒ. 36

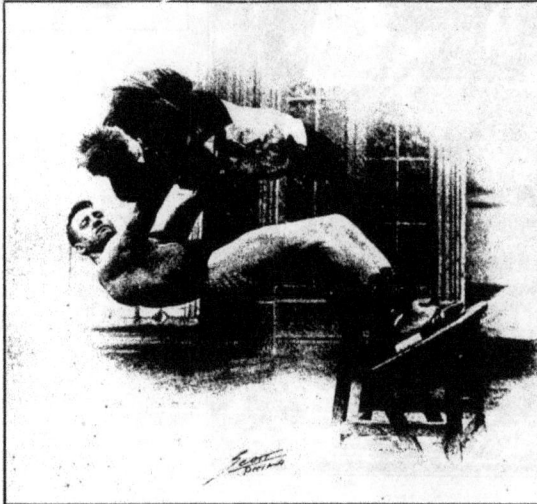

Plate 19, Figure 36 (a b o v e). Holding a light weight at the back of the neck, and coming to a sitting position to develop the muscles at the front of the abdomen

Fig. 40

Figure 40 (below). A feat of strength on a Roman Chair. This stunt requires g r e a t strength in the thighs and hips, as well as in the a b d o m i n a l muscles

PLATE 20

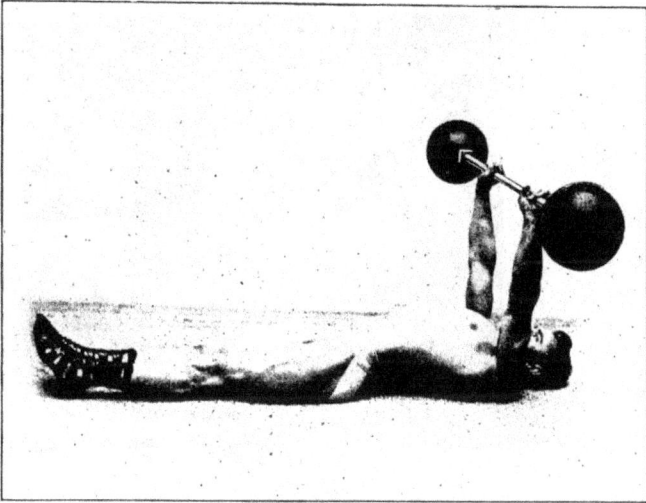

Fig. 41

Plate 20, Figure 41 (above), shows the start of the chest developing exercise

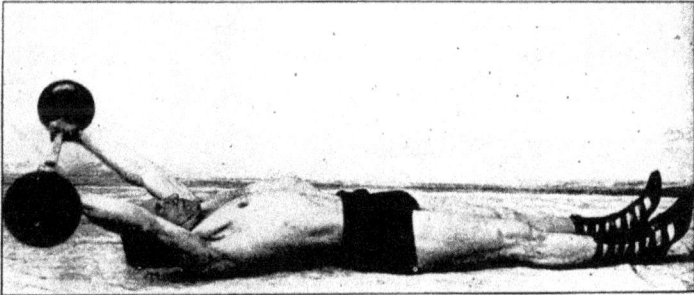

Fig. 42

Figure 42 (below), shows the bell part way down. Some men have increased the size of their chests 12 inches by specializing on this exercise, whcih is fully described in the text

PLATE 21

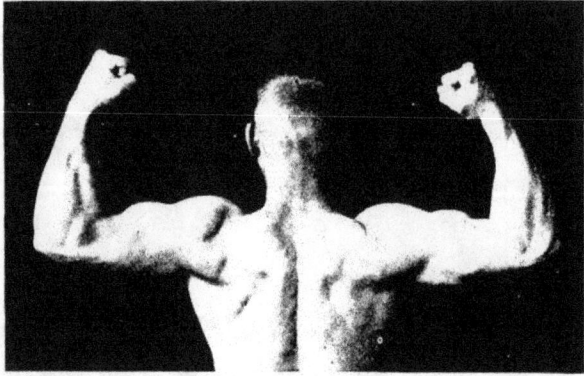

Fig. 43

Plate 21, Figure 43 (above). The usual and correct pose to display the muscles of the arms and upper back

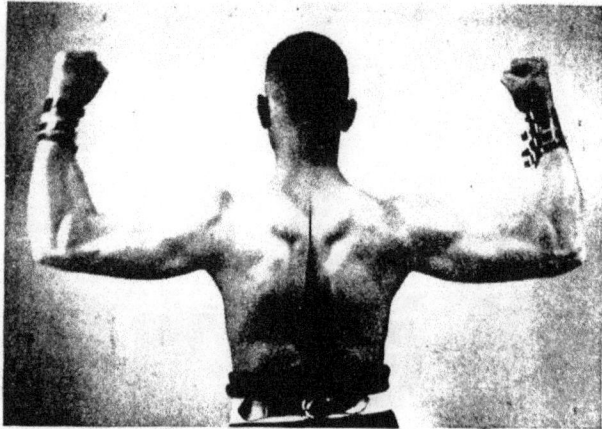

Fig. 44

Figure 44 (below). In this pose the athlete, by squeezing his shoulder blades together, has made his back narrower than it really is, although he manages to display more muscles in the center of the back

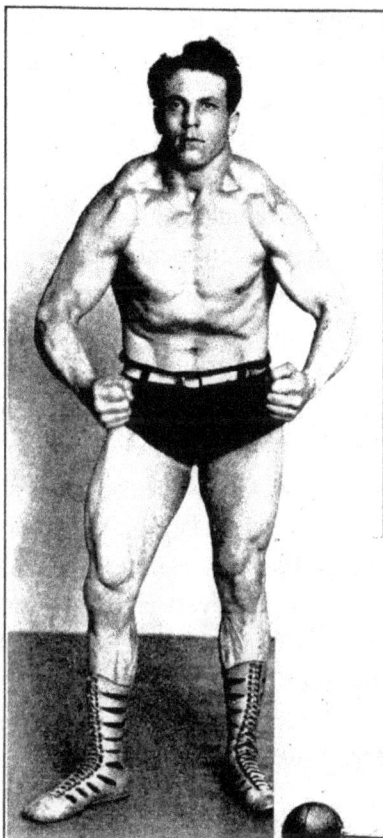

PLATE 22

Fig. 45

Plate 22, Figure 45 (above). Henry Steinborn posing in a way that shows the huge trapezius muscles, which lie on the upper part of the back, near the base of the neck. When the upper part of these muscles are flexed, they appear as two huge humps between the sides of the neck and the points of the shoulders.

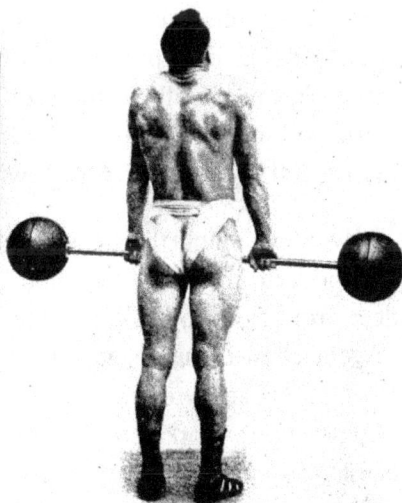

Fig. 46

Figure 46 (below), shows the shoulder shrugging exercise, which develops the trapezius muscles. After the shoulders have been shrugged, the shoulder blades should be pressed together. This makes the triceps muscles assume a basin-like shape, which can clearly be seen at the base of the neck in this pose.

79

The very best exercise for increasing the size of the rib-box is the following: Lie flat on the back; take a light bar-bell and pull it across the face to the chest; push it to arms' length, as in Fig. 41; and then, keeping the arms stiff and straight, you lower the bell in a quarter-circle movement until it rests on the floor at arms' length beyond the head. (Fig. 42 shows it part way down.) Still keeping the arms stiff and straight, you raise the bell again until it is above the chest. I have seen some men practise this exercise faithfully and get only a 2- or 3-inch increase in chest measurement; and I have seen others do it no oftener and get an increase of 8 or 9 inches. Prof. H. B. Lange, who had a 36-inch chest at the age of 30, has gotten his chest measurement up to more than 50 inches. Most of the increase he ascribes to intelligent practice of this exercise. Occasionally, when a student complains to me that while his strength is rapidly increasing, he is not gaining in size, I take him off all the other work and make him practise this exercise exclusively every day (and sometimes twice a day), for a period of, a month. I have seen men add 4 inches in one month to the size of their chests by this special work; and after they resumed their regular training program, the muscles all over their bodies grew in size at a surprising rate.

By developing the upper back muscles, anyone can add to the width of his chest. The important thing is to make your chest deep from front to back; and the thing which controls the depth of your chest is the distance between your breast-bone and your spine. You can by doing gymnastics, such as horizontal-bar and "Roman-ring" work, so develop the upper muscles that your chest will appear very wide; but even if you develop the big muscles on your breast, the upper part of your chest will still be flat. If, however, you increase the depth of your chest, the upper chest will become high-arched, and spring out in a swelling curve right from the base of the neck, the way it does in some of the Greek athletes whose statues you have seen.

There is an author by the name of Talbot Mundy who is very fond of introducing "Strong Men" into his stories. In his tales of India and the Far East, his Herculean character, Jeff Ramsden, is continually getting into personal combat with gigantic Arabs or East Indians. Mr. Mundy does not tell of professional "Strong Men" or vaudeville performers, but of natural "Strong Men"; and whenever he introduces such a character, he almost always says that the man in question has broad shoulders and is "ribbed-up like a race-horse." The minute you think of a race-horse, you get a picture in your mind of a slender-waisted animal with an enormously deep chest. If you could see the skeleton of a race-horse you'd notice that the rear-ribs are small and that each pair of ribs seems to get longer; until when you get to the front and longest pairs, the depth of the race-horse's chest is as great as that of a 2000-lb. truck horse. Now, if a man has a chest "like a race-horse," it means that the ribs which fasten to the breast-bone are unusually long, and that his chest is unusually deep from front to back. Mr. Mundy evidently knows the trade-marks of a natural "Strong Man," because he emphasizes the one great essential, and that is the rib-box which is deep from front to back.

Technically, this chest-exercise is known as the "two-arm pullover," which is rarely used as a competitive lift. Any man who can raise a 100-lb. bell from the floor to above his chest with straight arms, is very unusually strong. I have heard stories of men raising 150 lbs. in this way, but I have never seen anyone do more than 120 lbs. The correct thing for you to do is never to practice it as a lift, but as an exercise; (that is, until you have had many months' experience). If you spend your time in trying to see how much weight you can raise, you will spoil it as a developing exercise, because the developing effect comes mostly from the manner in which you lower the bell. If you fail to get results from practicing, the fault is not with the exercise but with you. In the first place, the arms must be stiff and straight, and that means that they must not be bent the least trifle at the elbows. I have seen men do the exercise with the arms slightly bent at the elbow; and because they didn't bend the arms any further while raising the bell, they would insist that their arms were straight. The moment you bend the arms at the elbow, you throw more work on are arm muscles and less on the muscles which control the ribs. The correct way is to lower the bell slowly; and as you lower it, you must take a deep breath and spread the ribs as far apart as possible. As you raise the bell, you breathe out. It is a vital mistake to use too much weight or to count the repetitions. The act of counting distracts your attention, which should be concentrated on the correct performance of the movement. You should lower and raise the bell as many times as you comfortably can. Another important detail is to keep the lower part of the spine as straight as possible. As you lower the bell you will feel a natural impulse to arch the lower part of the spine and to allow the small of the back to raise from the floor. The farther the lower back leaves the floor, the less the ribs will spread; so you must try to prevent your abdomen from rising in the air as you lower the bell.

If you weigh less than 135 lbs. and have had no experience, use a 25-lb., or even a 20-lb., bar-bell. If you weigh 150 lbs. and are in fair condition, use a 30-lb. bar-bell; and if you are a 200-lb. man, in good shape, you can use 40 or 45 lbs. I caution you against using a definite progressive schedule. It will be sufficient if you increase the weight of the bell 2½ lbs. a month; and I believe that 50 lbs. is enough for any man to use in this exercise for the purpose of chest development.

When I said above that you must take a deep breath as you lower the bell, I did not mean that you were to pack the lungs with air to such an extent that your eyes pop out and your face becomes red. The bell must be lowered slowly, but not very slowly. This stunt will give you a wonderful chest development if you follow the above directions.

Incidentally, the act of raising the bell will develop the muscles on inside of the upper-arms and those across the broad of the back; but that development is incidental. It is a "by-product," because the aim of the exercise is to add size and flexibility to the rib-box. You can get all the development you can possibly want on the outside of your chest by practicing the exercises for the arms, shoulders and upper back, which will be described in subsequent chapters.

CHAPTER IX

THE UPPER PART OF THE BACK

If you have been a steady reader of the magazines devoted to body-building, you must have noticed that they constantly publish pictures of athletes displaying the upper-back development; and that most of the athletes pose as in Fig. 43. There are two reasons for this. The first one is that when you raise the arms in that position, you can flex both the upper-arm and forearm muscles so as to make your arms look big from wrist to shoulder. The act of holding the upper arms horizontally makes the deltoid muscles flex in a pleasing manner. Another reason is that this is the accepted position for showing the muscles across the upper part of the back. It is easier to build muscles across the upper back than on almost any other part of the body. So most men who take up exercise show results there more quickly than in their arms and much sooner than in their legs. Again, upper-back exercises are so easy, and cause such little fatigue, that the beginner is tempted to spend all his time at such exercises. Many a man has had a reputation as a "Strong Man" because he shows up well when he has his picture taken in this pose; whereas, if he had a full-length back view taken, it would reveal that the lower part of his back, his haunches and his legs, showed no more development than that of the average 16-year-old boy. Understand me, upper-back development is important, but not nearly as important as development in the lower part of the back.

First, we will consider the trapezius muscles, which are situated along the upper third of the spine. The two muscles together look something like an old-fashioned kite. Their business is to raise, or shrug, the shoulders, or to pull the shoulder-blades closer together. When the vertical fibers of these muscles flex and pull the shoulder-blades together, the appearance is as in Fig. 44. When the upper fibers are flexed, the appearance is as in Fig. 45.

While everyone knows what is meant by "round shoulders," there are only a few who know what is meant by "square shoulders." Some people think that "square shoulders" mean that when you look at a man from the front, his shoulders go out in a straight line from the base of his neck; whereas, "square shoulders" are shoulders which are flat across the upper back. Well-posted novelists have a trick of saying, "His shoulders were sloping, as is the case in every real 'Strong Man.' " That is true enough. If viewed from the front, the line of the shoulders should slope from the sides of the neck downwards and outwards to near the points of the shoulders; and when this slope is pronounced, it means that the athlete has properly developed trapezius muscles.

The simplest way to develop the trapezius is to hold a fairly heavy bar-bell in the hands and shrug the shoulders, as in Fig. 46. The exercise is amazingly simple. Your arms are simply ropes which attach the weight to the shoulder muscles. Every time you shrug your shoulders the hands are lifted two or three inches, and after the shoulders are raised high as possible, you squeeze the shoulder-blades together. The trapezius muscles are very much stronger than their size would indicate. They are called into vigorous action every time you raise a weight from the ground. If you practice the Jefferson exercise, or a hand-and-thigh lift, the trapezius muscles are developed very rapidly. If you do a hand- and-thigh lift correctly, the only place you feel it is in these trapezius muscles and in the thighs. When you carry a very heavy weight in one hand, it is the trapezius that keeps your shoulder up. I have seen an athlete fasten one end of the chain to a 400-lb. weight, wrap the other end of the chain around his wrist, and then, while standing erect, raise the weight an inch from the floor just by shrugging the shoulder. Naturally, he gripped the chain with his hand, and the turns around his wrist were just to keep the chain from slipping out of his grasp. He stood straight-legged, and did not bend his arm at the elbow, and all the lifting-power came from the contraction of the right half of the trapezius muscle. The trapezius muscles and some of their smaller neighbors help to move or control the position of the shoulder-blades; and if the shoulder-blades protrude almost like sails, as they do in some people, I it means that those individuals have probably caused that condition by unconsciously hunching the shoulders in a way that makes certain muscles contract and lifts the shoulder-blades out of their normal position. I know bar-bell users who can do the most astonishing things in the way of controlling the appearance of their upper back. They can move their shoulder-blades around as easily as you would move your thumbs. They can raise the blades, lower them, and make them project or lie flat at will. Later on I will have a few words to say about the so-called "muscle control."

The biggest muscles in the back are called the "latissimus dorsi," which means the "broad of the back." Their main function is to pull the arm backwards and downwards; and, therefore you find these muscles highly developed in gymnasts who have done much work on the Roman-rings. These muscles, like all others, work in two different ways, depending on which end of the muscle is flexed for the time being. In climbing a rope, the forearm is the fixed point in this case, and the contraction of the latissimus dorsi muscle helps to pull the body up towards the forearm. On the contrary, if you are standing on the ground and pull downwards on the rope of a hand-power elevator, your body is the fixed point, and the contraction of the muscle pulls the forearm down to the body.

The next chance you get to watch a man pulling up a hand-power elevator, be careful to notice the way he does it. Any man who is not used to the job pulls entirely by arm strength, but a workman who does it every day bends his body forward from the hips with each downward pull of the arms. In this way he adds some of the weight of his upper body to supplement the strength of his arms. (You can get a lot of points on strength economy and muscular efficiency by watching the methods of men who earn their living by doing heavy labor.)

These latissimus dorsi muscles are so big that they control the shape of your sides. The side-line of the body from the arm-pit to just above the waist is dependent on the size and shape of your latissimus muscles, and the ultimate size of your chest is influenced by the development of these muscles and other muscles in the back. Suppose, for instance, that the pectoral muscles on your breast and the upper back are each one-half inch thick. By developing them to a point where each is one inch thick you add one inch to the diameter and, consequently, more than three inches to the circumference of your chest. I remember one authority on physical culture who said that, while he -acknowledged that the use of barbells and weights would develop all the muscles used in raising the weight from the ground, he did not see how, by using barbells, you could develop the muscles which would pull weights downward. (I suppose he meant the muscles you would use when pulling on the rope of a hand-power elevator, or in climbing a fixed rope.) In such stunts the work is done largely by the flexors of the arms (the muscles that bend the arms), and the muscles on the upper body which pull the arm downwards. When you lie flat on your back and do the two-arm pull-over, which was illustrated in Fig. 42, the work of raising the bell is done by the muscles just referred to. Steady practice of the chest-developing exercise would give you a fine pair of latissimus muscles; and if you wish to accentuate the development, all you have to do is to use a bell almost as heavy as you can raise with stiff arms, and repeat the lifting movement three or four times in succession. (You must not, however, use a heavy bell when you practice the two- arm pull-over as a chest-expanding exercise, because with a really heavy bell it is impossible to lower the arms as slowly as you should.)

You will find the latissimus muscles highly developed in most first-class oarsmen, and one of the best bar-bell exercises is somewhat like pulling on a pair of oars. You bend the body over at right angles, letting the bar-bell hang at arms' length, as in Fig. 47. Then you pull the bell up to your chest, as in Fig. 48. When raising the bell you should be careful to point the elbows outward, as well as upward, instead of bringing the elbows close to the side of the waist. The above exercise is for the beginner, and you can start with 20 or 30 lbs. and increase up to 75 or 80 lbs. That exercise is a favorite with German and Austrian lifters; but in my opinion it has a restricted value. One objection to it is that when the bar-bell gets heavy (more than half your own weight) you waste too much energy in trying to keep yourself from toppling over on your face. Another objection is that it does not give a full contraction of the back muscles, because the motion stops when the bar-bell handle touches your chest. It seems to me much better to use a kettle-bell or a dumbbell, and exercise one arm at a time. When you lean the body over at right angles, and rest one hand on the seat of a chair, then when you raise the kettle-bell in the other hand, you can bring the elbow of the lifting arm much higher, as in Fig. 49, and since the chair acts as a brace you can put a great deal more energy into the lifting movement. Also you can use very much heavier weights and get greater development without waste of energy. If you start with a 35-lb. kettle- bell, you will find that in a few weeks you can pull up 75 to 100 lbs. almost as easily, and that there will have been a great improvement in the development and the shape of your back.

There are a number of smaller muscles in the upper back, but the ones I have mentioned are the main muscles, and in working these main muscles you involve the smaller ones. If I had the space I would tell you all about the other back muscles, but if I once got started I would be apt to write on that subject to the end of the book.

CHAPTER X

THE SHOULDER MUSCLES

The true shoulder-muscles are the ones on the points of the shoulders which cover the shoulder-joint. These muscles are called the "deltoids," because they are triangular shaped like the Greek letter Delta. The base of the triangle is fastened to the bones which form the shoulder-girdle, and the point of the muscle is attached to the bone of the upper arm. When the muscle contracts it lifts the arm outwards and upwards. The anterior, (forward) set of fibers (that is, the fibers nearest the collar bone) lift the arm forwards and upwards; the lateral muscle-fibers lift the arms sideways and upwards, and the posterior fibers lift it backwards and upwards. The posterior fibers are brought into active play when you lift a kettle-bell, as in Fig. 49, and that exercise, which develops the latissimus muscle, also develops the back of your deltoid muscles.

Any time that you lift an object above your head you are giving your deltoids very vigorous work. In light-exercise courses the pupil is told to take a 5-lb. dumbbell in each hand; to stand with the arms hanging at the sides, and then raise the arms until they are level with the shoulders. Part of the time he is to lift the arms straight out in front of him, but most of the time he raises them sideways. These two movements leave the back of the deltoids untouched, and I think it was Prof. Barker who suggested that the body be inclined forward from the hips before lifting the bells sideways. This variation brings more of the muscle into play. The deltoids are so powerful that it takes more than 5-lb. weights to develop them. For some reason or other straight-arm raising is one of the most exhausting of all exercises, and when you use 10, 15 or 20 lbs. the work of raising the arms from the hang to the horizontal position is very tiring.

A much easier way to develop the deltoids is to practice lifting moderately heavy dumbbells or bar-bells to arms' length above the head; and if you use a dumbbell in a certain way you can get a most beautiful development of the deltoids. Ninety-nine men out of a hundred have the idea that when a "Strong Man" pushes a big dumbbell overhead the work is done entirely by the muscles of the upper arm, forgetting that, while the triceps muscles on the back of the upper arm will straighten the arm after it is bent, the actual work of raising the arm above the head is done by the deltoids. This explains why so many men with fine upper arms fail utterly when they try to push aloft even a moderately heavy weight. Every one of you is familiar with what we call the "floor-dip," where the athlete first assumes the position shown in Fig. 50, and while keeping his body rigidly straight, raises and lowers it by bending and straightening the arms. The average physical culturist, who can do this only three or four times when he first learns it, becomes able in a few months' practice to repeat it 30, 40, or even 50 times. By so doing he gets a fair development of the outer head of the triceps muscle, and a good development of the pectoral muscles on the breast, but hardly any development of the deltoids on the shoulders. When he is asked to take a 75-lb. dumbbell in his right hand and raise it to arms' length above the head he can't even start it on its upward journey away from the shoulder, and this puzzles him very much, because he knows that his upper arms are strong. He is still more surprised if he sees a workman, who has been accustomed to using a pick and shovel, push the dumbbell up fairly easily—especially if that workman happens to have an upper arm smaller than his own. The explanation is that every time the workman raises a pick-ax above his head he uses his deltoids, and every time he scoops up a shovelful of dirt and chucks that dirt onto a high pile, it is his deltoids which lift his arms. I hope eventually to convince you that his upper-arm muscles are the last thing a "Strong Man" worries about. He knows that if he fully develops the deltoids and the muscles on the upper body which control the movement of the whole arm, and if he develops the wrist and forearm to the full, his upper arm muscles will develop almost of their own accord, and will be equal to any demand he can put upon them.

If you take a moderately heavy bar-bell in your two hands, stand with your feet apart and well braced, keep your body upright, and push the bar-bell to arms' length several times in succession, as in Fig. 51, you will develop the triceps and deltoid muscles at the same time; but you will get more effect in the shoulder muscles than in the arm muscles. No one of you should go anywhere near the limit of your arm strength in this exercise until you have strengthened the lower back by practicing the exercises in Chapter II. An easier way to develop the deltoids is to use a pair of kettle-bells and to push the arms aloft one at a time, as in Fig. 52. As you raise the right arm you should lower the left arm, and at the completion of the movement, after the right arm has been straightened, you should reach up with the right shoulder and reach down as far as possible with the left elbow. When the left arm goes up and straightens you reach up with the left shoulder and down with the right elbow. This little extra motion at the end of the lift will add greatly to the strength and development of the shoulder muscles, and should not be omitted. If you start with 15 lbs. in each hand you can quickly work up until it is easy to do it with 40 lbs. in each hand. I have seen a professional start his work out by doing this exercise with 75 lbs. in each hand; and he did it not as a feat of strength but just as an exercise to warm up the shoulder muscles.

There is another and even better way of using a dumbbell for shoulder and upper back development. (The two things cannot be separated.) In your upper arm the biceps-flexor bends the arm, and it is opposed by the triceps which straightens or extends the arm. The deltoids and some of the back muscles oppose each other in the same way, and when you find a man with big, rounded muscles on the points of his shoulders you almost invariably find that that man has an equally remarkable development of the muscles of the upper back and broad of the back. (By the way, in our line of business the broad of the back does not mean the widest part of the back between the shoulders. The small of the back is that part of your back at your waist-line. The broad of the back is where the back starts, just above the waist, and spreads out to the arm pits. That part of the back above the arm pits is always alluded to as the shoulders, or the upper back. There is a great deal of difference between being broad backed and broad shouldered. A man with a big frame, but no muscular development, can have broad shoulders and yet, owing to lack of muscular development, be narrow in the broad of the back. The following exercise develops both shoulder and back muscles.

Take a 25-lb. dumbbell and lift it to your shoulder. Step forward with the left foot, which makes you stand about as in Fig. 53. Rest most of your weight on that advanced left foot; lean your body over in the direction to which the left toes point, and as you lean over push the bell to arm's length with the right arm. Straighten up, and, as you do so, lower the right arm slowly, so that when the arm is down the hand holding the bell will be just opposite the shoulder and about 8 inches away from the shoulder, as in Fig. 54. The arm must be lowered slowly, and as it is lowered you must deliberately harden the muscles on the right side of the upper back, so that the horizontal right upper arm will be supported on a shelf of muscle. If you get the trick correctly you will find that all you have to do is to again bear your weight on your left foot, bend your body over and the bell will go up almost of its own accord. You should use a bell of such weight that you can repeat the movement ten or twelve times. All the benefit comes from the way you do the exercise, and the weight used is of less importance. It is folly to use a 5- or 10-lb.dumbbell, because so little weight would throw no "developing strain" on the muscles. It is just as much of a mistake to use a bell which requires all your strength to put it aloft. If you think this is a "lift" and waste your time in seeing how much weight you can push to arm's length, the development you get will be very disappointing. If you use a moderate weight and do the exercise correctly you will get simply wonderful shoulder and back muscles. The back muscles are developed through the act of contracting them as you lower the arm. The deltoid is developed by the act of raising the bell, but even more by the way you lower the bell. In Fig. 54 the hand holding the bell is almost halfway to the muscled-out position. Practically every man can start this with 20 lbs. Others who are bigger and stronger can start with 25, 30, or 35 lbs. This movement develops the muscles so rapidly that it is possible to increase the weight of the bell a couple of pounds every week. If you are a light man 50 lbs. should be your limit; if you are a big man you can go as high as 65 lbs., but you must always keep firmly fixed in your head the idea that this is a developing exercise and is not a lift in any sense of the word. No man could make a big one-arm lift in this style, although it is almost the best possible training for some of the muscles used in overhead lifting.

Look at any illustrated book written by those travelers who have visited South Africa, the South Sea Islands or other parts of the globe where the natives wear but few clothes. In the photographs showing the natives you will see that all of the men have quite large pectoral or breast muscles, even though they show but little development in the arms. I have never been able to satisfactorily account for such development, because in civilized lands the only men who show that development are gymnasts. These same muscles are distinctly outlined in the old Greek statues. Some of the great "Strong Men" have highly developed pectoral muscles, but these muscles are not particularly noticeable, because they are accompanied by equal development in the neighboring part of the body. At present there seems to be a cult among physical culturists for development of the breast muscles. If you will turn to the various pictures of celebrated "Strong Men" which appear in this volume you will not find one man who shows anything abnormal in the way of breast-muscle development. If a man has big muscles on the upper front chest and little development elsewhere, naturally, these muscles will appear abnormally large, but if the shoulders are wide, the deltoids well developed, and the arms covered with muscle, then the pectorals don't seem nearly so big. In the picture of Sandow, Fig. 55, you can see pair of pectorals just as big as those of the average Zulu, but you don't notice these muscles unless you look for them, because they harmonize with the rest of his development. These pectoral muscles are not nearly as important as some of you think they are. Anyone who has spent a lot of time at the "floor-dip" or "dipping" on the parallel bars,

93

or who did Roman-ring work, is bound to have highly developed pectoral muscles, but the finest pectorals I ever saw on any man were on a weight-lifter who rarely practiced dipping. If he did the floor-dip at all he did it with his arms straight, holding them stretched out beyond the head or straight out to the sides. When you do the floor-dip with the arms straight, the chest can be raised only a few inches from the floor, and the work of raising the body is done by the muscles which control the arms. The pectorals get the hardest work in that variation of the floor-dip when the arms are stretched straight out to the sides. The lifter in question, instead of doing the floor-dip, would lie flat on his back with a 40-lb. dumbbell in each hand (Fig. 56), and spread his arms out to the sides, and while keeping the arms stiff and straight bring the hands together by lifting the arms. Few people can do this with 40 lbs., and 20 lbs. is enough for the average beginner to use at the start.

The pectoral muscles are not nearly as important as the muscles on the back, although they should not be neglected. It is a fatal mistake to try to increase the size of the chest just by thickening the pectoral muscles. Those muscles are fastened to the breastbone at one side and to the upper arm bone at the other, and so their tendency is to pull the shoulders forward and closer to the breast-bone; which explains why some of these parallel-bar specialists have become permanently round shouldered. Development on the front part of the chest must be balanced by even greater development on the upper back. This is another case where the mirror is to blame. The beginner will work like mad to develop the chest muscles, because he can see them in his mirror, just the same way that he develops the muscles on his abdomen and on the front and outside of his thighs. Because he cannot examine them with ease he neglects the far more important muscles on the upper back, the small of the back and the back of the legs. Man is an upright animal, and one of the main objects of training is to make the individual as

94

upright as possible. When you find a man who is possessed of super-strength, you find a man who is as "straight as an arrow."

All the muscles on the upper trunk, the pectorals, the deltoids, and the muscles across the back of the shoulders can be quickly and easily developed by what is called "straight-arm work," because when the arm is held straight all that the muscles on the upper arm do is to keep the arm in alignment, and the arm as a whole is moved to various directions by the contraction of the muscles which have their origin and base on the bones of the upper part of the trunk, and their attachments on the upper arm bone. The exercise in Fig. 42 develops the back muscles, because the arms are held straight as you lift the bell. In the ordinary shoulder exercise the arms are likewise held straight, and the same thing is true of the chest exercise, Fig. 56.

One of the greatest strength stunts on a pair of Roman rings is for the athlete to hold himself in the position known as "the cross," with one ring is each hand, the arms held straight out to the sides and the body upright. This is possible only for those men who have great strength in the upper body muscles. It is not hard to keep the arms straight, but it requires a great exertion to keep the body from immediately falling down so that the athlete is hanging by the hands. To maintain the "cross" position it is necessary to press downwards against the rings, and if you have read the text carefully up to this point I do not have to tell you that the muscles which enable you to press down with the hands are the ones on the broad of the back. (A lesser working strain is thrown on the deltoids and the pectorals.) This stunt is easy for a man with a powerful upper body and small lower limbs, while it is very difficult for a big 200-lb. man who is fully developed from head to foot.

A man who can do "the cross" on the rings may be able to "muscle-out" quite a heavy weight in each hand, although it is

95

quite likely that he cannot muscle-out an even heavier weight in one hand.

Fig. 57 shows what the English lifters call "the crucifix lift," and which the European lifters call "holding in the balance." One of the most popular of all strength tests is to hold a weight straight out from the shoulder in one hand; and it is a common thing to see a group of workmen or athletes in an impromptu competition with the object of seeing which one of them can "muscle-out" the heaviest weight. In some parts of this country they allude to this stunt as "off-arming." No matter what you call it, it is a fine test of strength, because anyone can do it without practice, there being little skill required. The proper way to "muscle-out" a weight is the European style, where you hold the weight by the ring with the knuckles of the hand up. You can do more if you hold the bell straight out in front of you, and while the athlete is allowed to advance one foot he is forbidden to lean back from the waist. If the average man does 25 lbs. in this style he is lucky. Any man who has practiced lifting bar-bells overhead has thereby developed such strength that he can muscle-out 40 or 50 lbs. at the first attempt. Bodily weight is a decided advantage and most of the records are held by big men. In France and Belgium, where this stunt is very popular, there are a number of athletes who have muscled-out between 80 and 90 lbs., but the record (112 pounds) was made by a German named Michael Meyer. (The old-timer, Carl Abs, is unofficially credited with 110 lbs.) Under the European rules the lifter does not raise the weight with a straight arm, but he lifts it with a bent arm until the weight is hanging right in front of the left shoulder, as in Fig. 58. Then he extends the right arm which holds the weight straight out in front of him, as in Fig. 59. When doing this stunt with a really heavy weight, there is an almost irresistible tendency to lean back from the waist in order to balance the weight; and this must be avoided, because as soon as you lean back, while your arm may be horizontal, it is no longer perpendicular to your body; whereas if you stand upright the body and arm are at right angles. If you and your friends have ever tried holding out a weight it is probable that you pushed the weight to arms' length over the head and then lowered the arm to the side with the weight resting on the palm of the hand, which is a perfectly admissible style, providing you keep the body upright and have the arm absolutely straight. A bunch of young huskies who are not acquainted with the rules are apt to hold the lifting arm slightly bent at the elbow, and to lean the body to the side in an effort to balance the weight, as in Fig. 60. In this lift the correct style is shown in Fig. 61. I have never seen more than 85 lbs. held out correctly at the side in one hand, although I have seen an athlete hold out correctly 80 lbs. in each hand. (There is a legend to the effect that the gigantic Louis Cyr once muscled-out a 135-lb. dumbbell; but I am quite sure that if this is true he must have broken the rules.) When you do muscle-out a bell to the side with the palm up, you're apt to feel a sharp pain at the lower end of the biceps, right on the inside of the elbow-joint; whereas if you're holding a weight out in front with the knuckles up there is no pain whatever.

Holding out one weight in each hand is in some ways easier than holding out a weight in one hand, because the two weights balance each other, and that is especially true if an illegal style is used. To take a 65-lb. dumbbell in each hand, "curl" the weights to the shoulders, push them aloft and then lower them with absolutely straight arms, as the position shown in Fig. 57, is a feat which requires tremendous strength in the arms and shoulders. Hackenschmidt is said to have done this with 90 lbs. in the right hand and 89 lbs. in the left hand, and the Russian lifter, Khryloff, did it with 90 lbs. in each hand; and Khryloff, if I can judge by his pictures, has the most magnificent-looking arm on record. There is an illegal method in which after the weights have been pushed aloft the arms are bent slightly at the elbow, and then the hands are lowered outwards until they are level with the top of the head. While holding the bells in this position the lifter bends his body backwards at the waist and rotates the hands until the palms are pointing to the rear of him. In this attitude the arm and shoulder muscles are "locked" in a sort of mechanical way, and because the lifter is leaning so far backwards a spectator standing in front of him gets the impression that the bells have been lowered as far as the shoulder-level.

In 1916 I saw a 145-lb. wrestler take in his right hand an 81-lb. dumbbell, and in the left hand a 79-lb. dumbbell, and do this stunt so cleverly that some of the spectators thought he was making an actual crucifix lift. This particular athlete had trained for years with bar-bells and was very clever in handling them. His flesh was of an extremely tough variety and he was almost insensible to pain; which was a good thing, because otherwise he could not have borne the strain of holding out the weights in the way he did. The two bells together weighed 15 lbs. more than he did himself; whereas no man had ever been able to properly hold out two dumbbells whose combined weight equaled his own. I doubt whether this man could have correctly held out more than 55 lbs. in each hand. The act of holding bells at arms' length; that is, of "muscling them out," is a feat of super-strength or a test of super-strength, but not a developing exercise. The exercises in the first part of this chapter, where you raise a weight, develop the shoulder strength which will enable you to "muscle-out" big weights.

PLATE 23

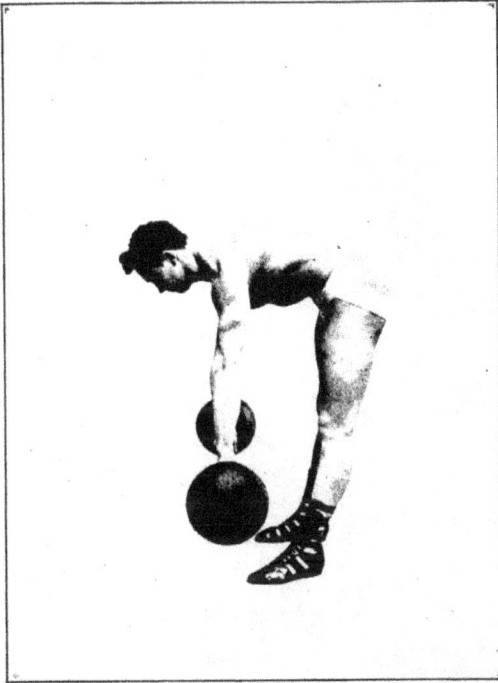

Fig 47

Plate 23. An
exercise to de-
v e l o p   t h e
muscles across
the broad of the
b a c k. S t a n d
straight - legged,
bend the body
at right angles,
as in Figure 47
(above), w i t h
bell hanging at
full length of
arms.

Fig. 48

Without moving the body or
legs, lift the bell by bending the
arms until the handle-bar
touches the chest, as in Figure
48 (below). Repeat several
times in succession. In this
exercise the elbows must be
pointed outwards, and raised as
high as possible. Do not let
the elbows come down by the
sides of the waist, as this will
bring the handle-bar across the
abdomen instead of across the
chest.

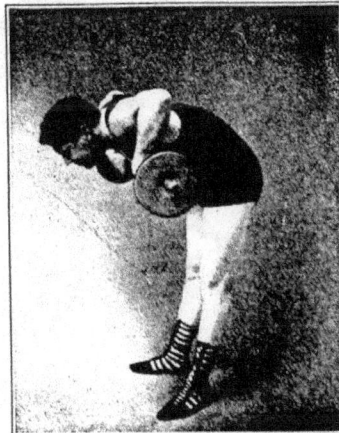

99

PLATE 24

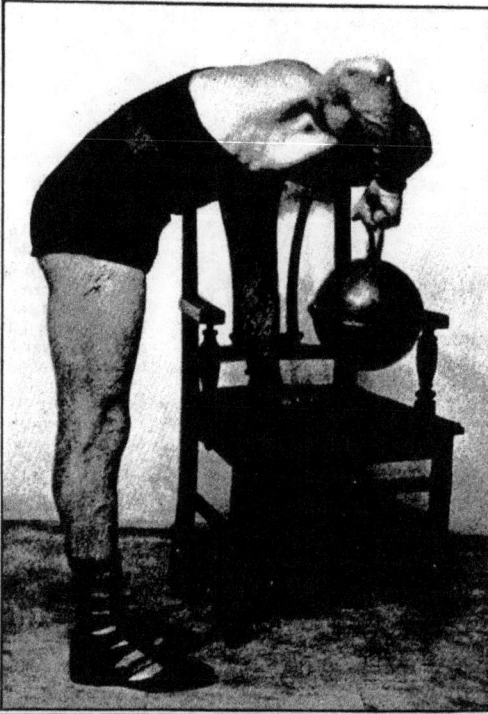

Fig. 49

Plate 24, Figure 49 (above), illustrates an exercise which is unequaled for developing the muscles on the broad of the back, and on the inside of the upper arm.

Fig. 50

Figure 50 (below), shows the ordinary "Floor Dip," which develops the back of the upper arms.

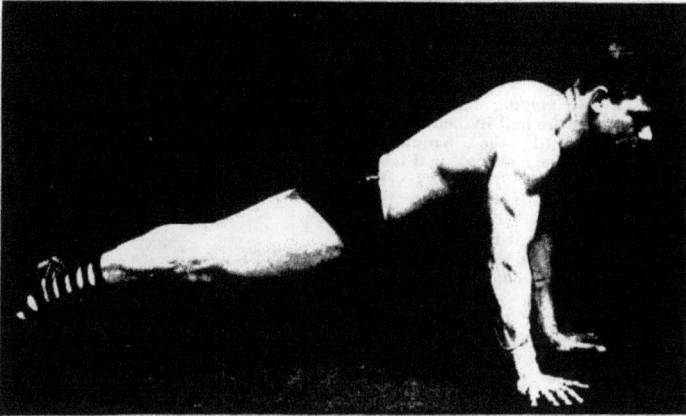

PLATE 25

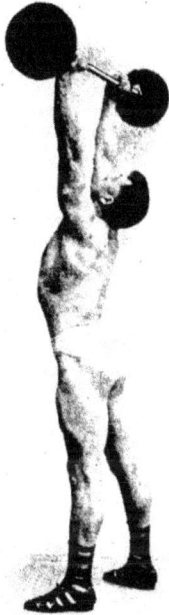

Fig. 51

Plate 25, Figure 51 (above), shows the ordinary "Two-Arm Press" with a bar-bell; which develops the deltoid muscles on the shoulders even more than it develops the pushing muscles of the arms

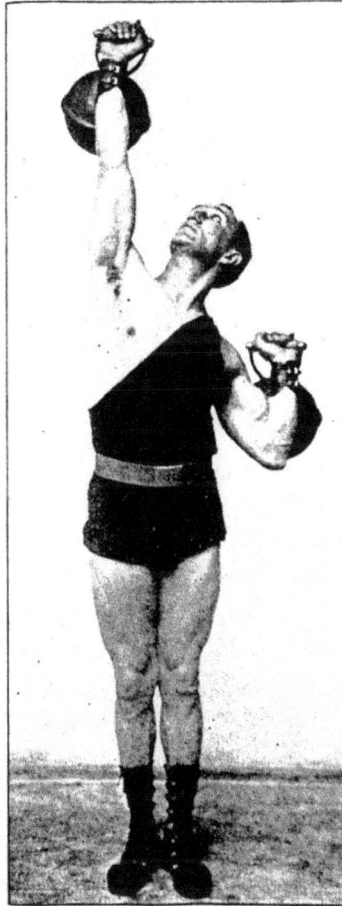

Fig. 52

Figure 52 (below), shows an exercise with two kettle-bells, which strengthens the arms and shoulders even more rapidly than does the two-arm "Press," shown in Figure 51. No one should work to his limit in the "two-arm press" until he has first strengthened his back by the exercises described in chapters 2 and 4

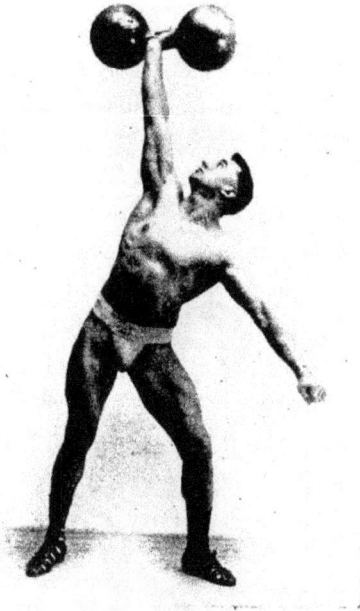

PLATE 26

Fig. 53

Plate 26, Figures 53 and 54, show an exercise which rapidly develops the shoulders and the upper back. In this exercise a moderate weight must be used, because the developing effect comes from the manner in which the lifting arm is lowered. After the bell has been once pushed to arms' length, as in Figure 53, the arm must be lowered slowly, and at the same time drawn slightly backwards. As the arm comes down, the muscles on the right side of the upper back should be hardened by an effort of the will.

Fig. 54

The bell must not be lowered further than shown in Figure 54. and the hand must be kept several inches from the shoulder. If the bell has been lowered correctly, all you have to do is to lean the body to the left, and the bell will go up almost of its own accord.

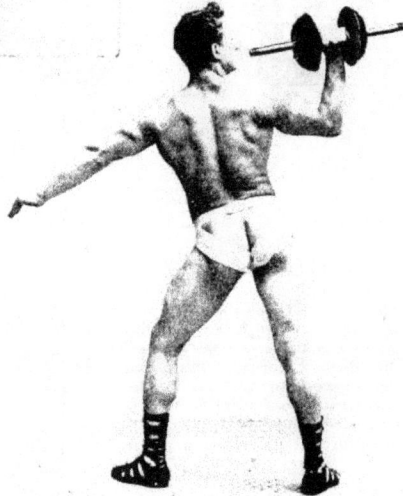

PLATE 27

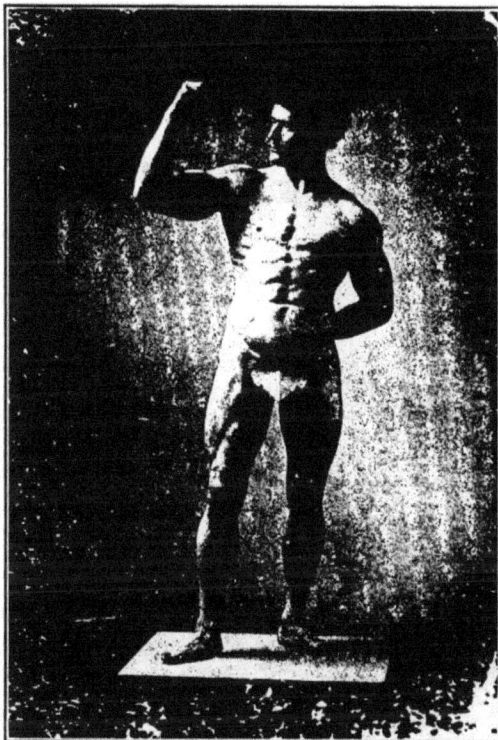

Fig. 55

Plate 27, Figure 55
(above). A pose by
Eugene Sandow, show-
ing that while his
breast muscles were
of unusual size, they
were not unduly
prominent, because
of the great size of
his shoulder and up-
per - back muscles.
Figure 56 (below).
An exercise which
develops the breast
muscles

Fig. 56

(Plate 27, Figure
56.) The arms are
kept perfectly
straight, and the
hands are raised un-
til they meet above
the chest. In this
picture the athlete is
using a pair of 15-lb.
dumbbells, and even
that light weight is
sufficient to cause a
marked contraction
of the breast muscles

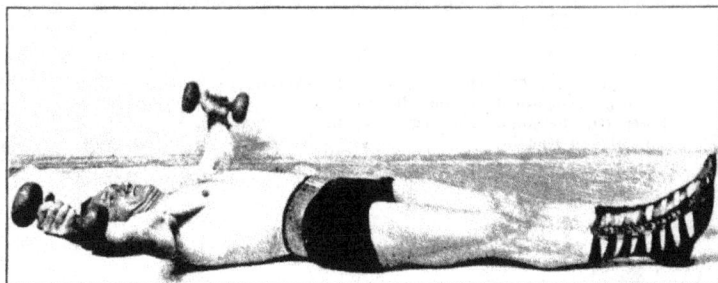

103

PLATE 28

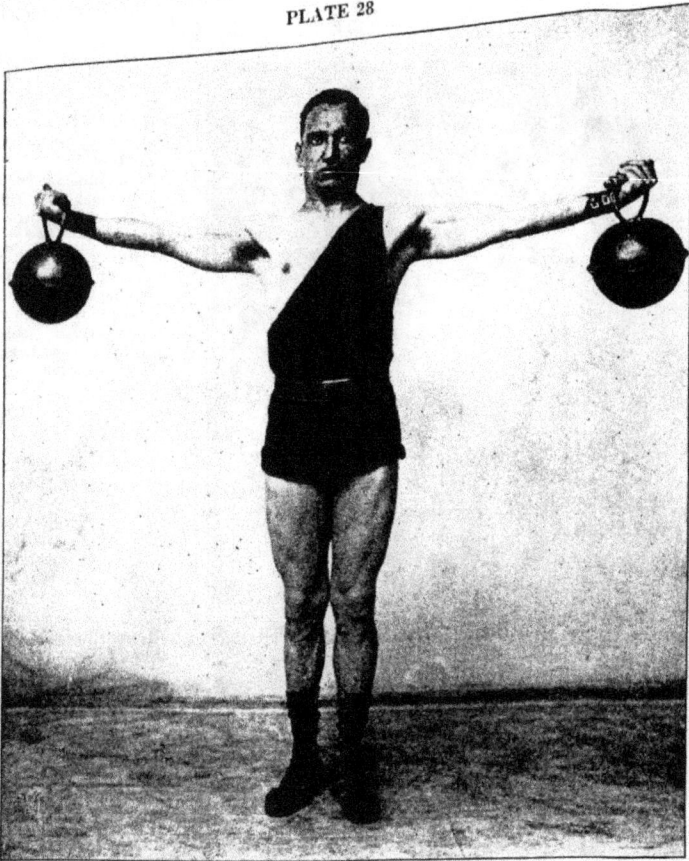

Fig. 57

Plate 28, Figure 57. The "Crucifix" lift correctly performed. After the bells are pushed to arms' length above the head, the arms are lowered to the sides. The arms must not be bent, and it is against the rules to lean backwards. You can add several pounds to your record in this lift if you put the handles of the dumbbells or the kettle-bells diagonally across the palms of the hands, as Mr. Donald is doing

PLATE 29

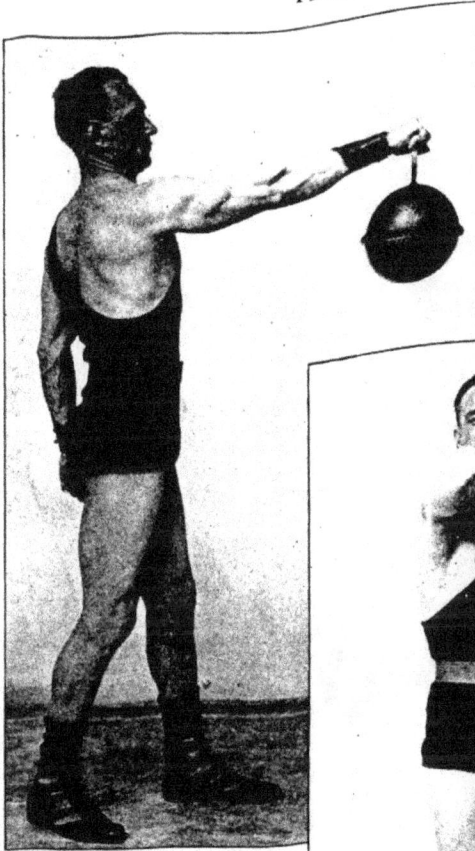

Fig. 58

Plate 29, Figure 58 (below), shows the start of the correct one-arm "Hold-out."

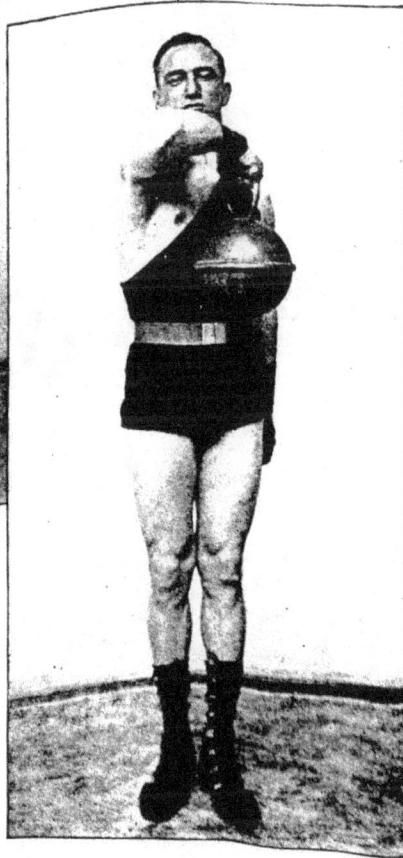

Fig. 59

Figure 59 (above), shows the finish of the lift. The body must be erect, the arm horizontal and rigidly straight, and the knuckles upward.

105

PLATE 30

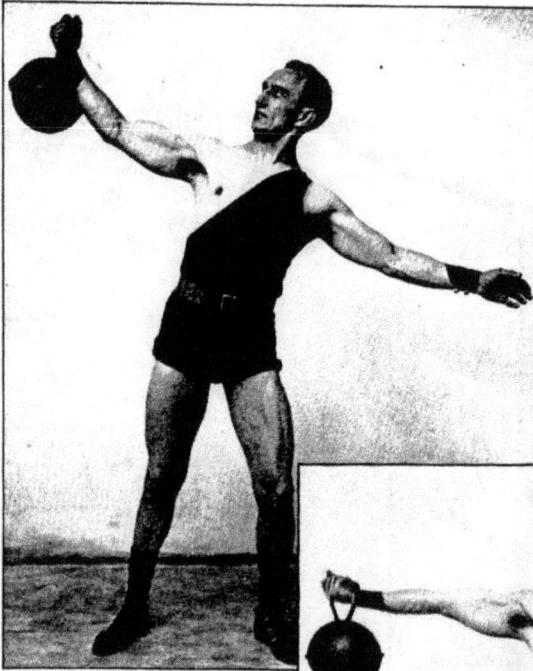

Plate 30, Figure 60 (a b o v e), shows the incorrect method of "Muscling - out" a w e i g h t, in which the arm has not been s t r a i ghtened, and the bell lowered o n l y part way

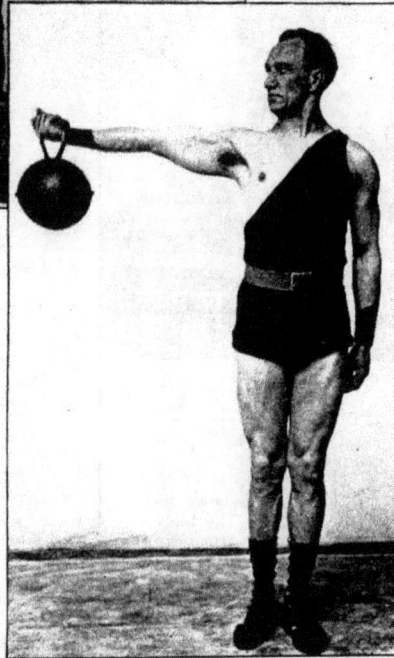

Fig. 61

Figure 61 (below), shows the correct method. The body must be upright, and the arm horizontal and p e r f e c t l y straight. Go easy on this lift at first, because if you use a too-heavy weight, you will feel a sharp pain at the lower end of the biceps muscle

CHAPTER XI

THE "SWING" AND THE "SNATCH"

So far I have said practically nothing about the upper arms, and have mentioned the arm muscles only incidentally, as they were involved in chest or shoulder-developing exercises. I did this deliberately with the attempt to make you realize the greater importance of back and leg strength to the super-strong man. Suppose we now analyze one lift in which a dumbbell is lifted to arms' length above the head in order that you may see how, in that lift, the bulk of the work is done by the shoulders, back and legs, and only a small part of the work done by the upper arm muscles.

In this lift, which is called the "one-arm swing," it is best to use a dumbbell. You stand with the feet apart and well braced with the dumbbell parallel to the feet, and the rear sphere a couple of inches beyond the toes. You lean over by inclining the body forward from the hips and by bending at the knees. Gripping the dumbbell with your hand close to the front sphere you lift it from the floor and swing it back between the legs—as in Fig. 62— keeping the arm straight.

This is simply to give you a start, because after the bell has reached the position in Fig. 62 you swing it forward again (keeping the right arm straight) in a semicircular movement until the hand which holds the bell is above your head. This is only a general description. What actually happens is that when the bell is opposite your eyes you quickly bend your knees and sit on your heels (as in Fig. 63), thus lowering your body in a way which enables you to get underneath the mounting bell. If you omit this second dip of the legs you will raise anywhere from 40 to 80 lbs. less than if you do use the legs correctly. If you will compare Fig. 62, showing the position at the commencement of the upward swing, with Fig. 12 in the chapter about back exercises, it will be seen that the positions are practically identical. The amount of vigor which you can put into swinging the bell forward and upward depends on the power with which you can press against the floor with your feet, and the vigor with which you can bring the body to the erect position. The more time you have spent in practicing the back and leg exercises, the more weight you will be able to "swing" aloft.

The arm movement, which is forward and upward, is caused by the vigorous contraction of the muscles on the shoulder and upper back; therefore, exercises like the one illustrated in Fig. 12, which develop the shoulder, also give you the kind of strength you need in this one-arm swing. In the chapter on leg exercises you were advised to practice constantly the exercise illustrated in Fig. 28, because that particular exercise not only developed the muscles in the thighs, but gave you the confidence necessary to sit on the heels while holding a weight at arm's length overhead. Unless you have practiced that exercise diligently you will find that you have not the confidence necessary to successfully complete a one-arm swing. There are lots of fine points about this lift; as for instance the pressing against the left thigh with the left hand which gives you a brace and assists you in straightening the body. There are a lot of details about "timing"—which is the art of selecting the exact fraction of a second when the bell has lost the impetus given it by the act of straightening the body and legs, and at which instant it is necessary to lower the body by the second bend of the knees. Some lifters at the start of the swing place the bell on the floor behind them and dispense with the preliminary backward swing. Some lifters bend the body sideways instead of straight downwards at the completion of the lift.

But it is not the aim of this book to give instructions in scientific lifting. Its object is to show you how to get more strength and to tell you about what constitutes real strength. It is necessary to tell you something about the technique of the lifts so that you can understand why it is that some of these skillful experts are able to lift such enormous weights. It is perfectly possible for you to get a beautifully proportioned and magnificently developed body without ever practicing any of what we call "the standard lifts," but it is very likely that after you have developed super- strength you will like to occasionally make a test to know how you compare with others; and such a test would be greatly to your disadvantage if you did not employ the methods which skilled lifters employ.

In the old times a man who attempted the swing would stand with his legs almost straight, and bend over by arching his back. He would by a tremendous effort swing the bell at arm's length above his head, and would not employ the second bend of the legs as modern lifters do. Consequently, even the biggest and strongest old-timers could not do more than 125 lbs. in the one-arm swing; whereas modern lifters do a great deal more than that. The old-time lifter was considered good if he could make a one- arm swing with a dumbbell which weighed a little more than half as much as he did himself; while the aim of a modern lifter is to make a one-arm swing with a dumbbell of his own weight. The world's record (so far as I know) is 199 lbs., which was accomplished by the French lifter, Jean Francois (Fig. 64). Several professionals and a few amateurs have swung over 190 lbs., and 175 to 180 lbs. is nothing extraordinary for a big man to swing. I have never yet seen or heard of a big man swinging a dumbbell of his own weight, although the feat has been accomplished by several small men. I believe that Thos. Inch, of London, weighing 160 lbs., did a one-arm swing with 160½ lbs. The present English record in the heavy-weight class is the 170-lb. lift of Edward Aston, and I believe that Aston himself does not weigh much more than that.

To successfully perform a one-arm swing with a bell almost as heavy as you are requires great speed of movement and accurate muscular co-ordination, as well as great bodily strength. To be successful in the quick lifts; such as the swing, the snatch and the jerk, you must have the speed of movement and the clever footwork of a boxer.

The point to be particularly noted is that when you perform a one-arm swing you do not feel the arm muscles working. The arm itself is held straight (though not rigid) throughout the entire lift, and it is just the part of you that transmits to the bell the power exerted by the contraction of the leg, back and shoulder muscles. If you use a moderate weight and perform a one-arm swing several times in succession, you get a fine exercise and one which will be valuable in teaching you co-ordination. It is necessary to learn all these "quick lifts" with a bell of such weight that you can handle it easily; but once you have mastered the principle governing the lift you will be able to increase the weight used very rapidly. In this one-arm swing you will probably be able to increase your record one hundred per cent within a few weeks after you do learn the methods, providing you have properly trained your back and legs. The advantage of making several successive lifts with a moderate weight is that the beginner always has a tendency to use too much arm strength and to try to finish the movement by an arm push. When making several repetitions the beginner's arm will tire rapidly, and about the third repetition he will find that, unconsciously, he is bending his knees more, and thus getting under the bell by lowering the body instead of by pushing with the arm. The more tired his arm gets the more he will bend his legs, and after a little experience of this kind he will be wise enough to do the second bend of the knees properly every time he swings the bell aloft. (Note: It is possible to use a kettle- bell instead of a dumbbell in the one-arm swing, but when using a kettle-bell you have to rotate the arm when the bell is opposite your face, so as to make the bell swing around and land on the back of the forearm, as in Fig. 65 (Frontispiece). This is a complicated motion that can be learned only by practice. If you do not rotate the arm correctly the kettle-bell will land against the upper arm with a jar that might break a bone. Since you can swing more weight in the shape of a dumbbell than in the shape of a kettle-bell it is hardly worth the bother to learn the method of using a kettle-bell. Sandow made a one-arm swing with a kettle-bell weighing, I think, 173 lbs. (I never heard his record with the dumbbell, but I am sure that he could swing a 190-lb. dumbbell.)

A somewhat similar and more popular lift is known as the "one-arm snatch," in which a bar-bell is used. The lifter stands back of the bell with the handle touching his ankles, leans over by bending the knees and inclining the body forward from the hips. In this lift you don't bend as far as you do in the one-arm swing and, therefore, it is necessary to round the back slightly. The bell is supposed to be pulled straight upwards in one unbroken line until it is at arm's length above the head, but most lifters raise the bell slightly forward as well as upward. In the one- arm swing the lifting arm is held straight throughout the entire performance of the lift, but in the one-arm snatch the arm is bent almost double when the bell is opposite the face. Just the same as in the swing, the lifter gets under the bell by lowering the body, and the correct instant at which to make the shift is when the bell has reached the level of the eyes. At the start of the snatch you stand up quickly, which means that you press hard against the floor with the feet, and straighten the legs and back at the same time; and if the movement is done correctly the bell will almost fly from the floor until it is opposite the chest. Continued practice is needed before you can exert sufficient power to make it fly up as high as the eyes. When the bell is that high you loosen your grip on the handle bar and instantaneously sit on your heels by bending the legs. This has to be done so quickly that you are under the bell with a straight arm, as in Fig. 66, before the bell has had time to drop an inch.

In the old times 100 lbs. was a good record in the snatch lift, because the lifters tried to throw the bell aloft solely by back and arm strength. The present record is somewhere between 215 and 220 lbs. Three years ago I erroneously stated that Henry Steinborn had created a new record when he made a one-arm snatch in Philadelphia with 208 lbs. I thought that the best previous lift was Vasseur's 205 lbs. I find that Vasseur has done close to 220 lbs. The night that Steinborn made his American record he had a few minutes before just barely failed to snatch 215½ lbs.

One of the most important parts of the snatch lift is where you ease up on your grip at the instant when you're getting under the bell, and in some cases they have gotten over his difficulty by using plate bar-bells in which the plates revolve very easily. Steinborn made his lift with the bell shown in Fig. 23. The plates fitted snugly over sleeves, which, in turn, fitted over the handle bar of the bar-bell. Between the sleeves and the bar there was a coating of vaseline; consequently the sleeves and plates would rotate very easily on the bar, making it unnecessary for Steinborn to loosen his grip. The night he made his record he snatched 208 lbs., and I know he could have done 220 in a one-arm snatch if that had been the only lift on the program. He did not push himself in the snatch, which was the first lift of the evening, because he was anxious, later on, to break Cyr's record in the two-arm "clean and jerk"; which he did.

I was told that Steinborn had a special bar constructed in which the sleeves revolved on ball bearings fitted between them and the bar. He came to me several days after he made his records, and when I told him I had found that Vasseur had done nearly 220 lbs. he wanted to make a bet with me that he could

112

beat anything Vasseur did. He told me that he would try for a new record in the one-arm snatch, and if I would give him $100 for every pound over 230, he would give me $10 for every pound under 230 if he failed to reach that mark. As I had seen the man do over 220 in practice, and knew what he could do (especially if he trained for one particular lift), I declined the bet and saved my money. This man, although very powerfully made, was as quick on his feet as Benny Leonard, or any light-weight boxer. The records in all quick lifts are at his mercy. When, to his prodigious strength, he adds his speed of movement and his sense of timing, he can transmit to a bar-bell an incredible momentum. (By the way, when he does the snatch he uses a peculiar grip. Instead of holding the bell with the thumb outside the fingers he bends his thumb and puts it in under the center of the bar and holds it there by placing the fingers outside of it. He claims that this makes it easier for him to make the "shift.")

In mentioning the records I have had to give those of the European lifters. This positively does not mean that the Europeans are any stronger than the men of this country. In Europe they have used bar-bells for years and competitive weight-lifting is a major sport. Consequently, the European lifters have, by the use of bar-bells, developed enormous strength and, by frequent competitive work, learned all the niceties of style. We, in this country, can do the same thing; in fact, we have done the same thing. Arthur Gildroy, who weighs 135 lbs., has made a one- arm snatch with 146 lbs., and the other American lifters who have specialized on the snatch-lifting have done practically as well as the foreign lifters. There is no country of its size which produces as many really "Strong Men" as does this country. The Dominion of Quebec, in Canada, produces natural "Strong Men" in wholesale quantities. In Finland they breed enormous men; but both Quebec and Finland are comparatively small, while this country is big. We have such an abundance of high-grade raw material that if we cared to go into competitive lifting I believe that America would hold the world's supremacy in that sport, just as it does in most other sports.

I have a friend in Philadelphia by the name of Jas. B. Juvenal, an ex-champion oarsman. From the time he was sixteen, Juvenal owned and used a 75-lb. dumbbell and a 150-lb. barbell. He had no adjustable bells because they were hard to get when he was a boy. He kept these bells at his boat club, and one day when he went to practice with them they were missing. The janitor said that he had been ordered by the captain of the club to throw the bells into the river. Juvenal hunted up the captain and gave his orders that the bells should be fished up again. As his reason for disposing of the bells the captain said that he was afraid that some of the younger club members would start exercising with them, and in that way get "stiff and muscle-bound." Whereupon, Juvenal stated that he had been using those bells for a dozen years, and that in all that time no man out of the hundreds who rowed on that river had been able to keep abreast of him—much less beat him—and that by using the bar-bells he had vastly increased his muscular power and never lost a bit of his speed of movement. This Mr. Juvenal is so strong that when we once held a competition at the "one-arm pull-over" the only man who could beat him was the famous Joe Nordquest; Juvenal took second place over a lot of celebrated "Strong Men." I once asked him to try a one-arm snatch with a 135-lb. bar-bell. This bell was a solid affair with a handle bar 1¾ inches thick. Juvenal made the lift, but it was not a true snatch. He actually made a back-handed swing with the bar-bell; that is, he kept his arm straight just as though he were swinging a dumbbell. If he had used a thin- handled bar-bell and known the correct way to snatch the bell, he could easily have done 180 to 190 lbs., as he weighed over 200 lbs. himself. Although he must be over 50 years of age I know that he could make an American amateur record in the snatch if he were enough interested to practice the method.

In concluding this chapter I wish to say that I have never seen a star at the snatch or swing who was not beautifully built. The top-heavy man—the man with big shoulders and thin legs—falls down utterly when he is asked to "swing" or "snatch" a really heavy weight. The men who hold the records in the swing and snatch are beautifully made. Their proportions are admirable, and they are of surpassing symmetry. Since the "quick lifts" require bodily strength it means that to succeed at these lifts you must have a body which is developed from head to heel.

But don't let us forget to analyze the action of the arm in the one-arm snatch. Because the weight is pulled almost directly upward the arm has to be bent as the bell mounts. When you first take hold of the bar the arm is straight and the knuckles of the hand are forward. (It would be impossible to make a snatch if you held the hand with the palm forward.) Therefore, the action of the arm is just the same as in the exercise for the upper back, illustrated in Fig. 49; and that, by the way, is the reason I described that exercise before I described the snatch lift. After the bell has reached the height of the face and you make the shift, the arm muscles are used hardly at all; because, if you bend your knees quick enough and far enough, your haunches will drop so far that you can get your body straight up and down, and your lifting-arm straight up and down under the bell. Then all you have to do is to stand erect to complete the lift. Here is another reason for practicing the exercise shown in Fig. 28.

Now let us go back to Mr. Juvenal. When he was in his racing shell and started a stroke, his body was bent forward almost double, and his knees against his chest; and as he made the stroke he straightened his legs, drew his body backwards and pulled his hands straight in; using the same muscles as you would use in a snatch lift. I understand that he could put such immense power into his stroke that he never was beaten in a quarter-mile sprint rowing race, and so it is no wonder that he is able to make a fine record in a one-arm snatch. Also it will be noted that as a young man he claimed the world's championship in the stunt where you sit down facing another man, and both of you pull on a broom handle. The winner is the man that pulls the other man off the floor. In this stunt one competitor presses the soles of his feet against the feet of the other man; and, as it is necessary to bend the knees slightly so as to lean forward and grasp the broom handle, the position is very much the same as at the beginning of the stroke in rowing. (I said "broom handle," but in lumber camps they use an ax handle. A broom handle would not last very long when gripped by two men of gigantic strength.) Once again let me say that I have found oarsmen to be far above the average in strength, especially those oarsmen who have devoted a lot of time to single sculling. They are an erect, square-shouldered, flat-back crowd, and their rowing has developed in them a keen sense of co-ordination. Almost any oarsman can be developed into a fine bar-bell lifter and can, if he cares to, greatly improve his physique by using bar-bells. He starts out with the advantage of knowing that it is important to know how to apply his strength. Juvenal, whose shoulders are immensely broad, has a chest of unusual depth. When he lies flat on his back and does the chest- developing exercises (Fig. 42) his chest swells up almost like a balloon as he lowers the bell.

CHAPTER XII

THE JERK LIFT

I am hurrying to get through with the technical descriptions of the various standard lifts, because I wish to get down to the really important part of this book; and that is the function of the barbell as a body-building and muscle-developing instrument. I used to be very fond of lifting, and made a study of it. I am still interested in it, and, consequently, when I write in these chapters about a certain lift I find that after I say, "In conclusion " I am apt a little later to say, "Finally" and still later, "Now just one word more" in the manner of all the other long-winded preachers. (I did it in the last chapter, and at that, I forgot to tell you there was a lift known as the two-arm snatch. It is just the same as the one-arm snatch except that you use two arms. To me it is a very unimportant lift, because it is a movement which you would rarely duplicate either in any kind of sport or in any kind of work.)

Next in order of discussion comes the lift known as "the jerk."In this lift, with the bell held at the height of the shoulders, the lifter (as in Fig. 67), while keeping his body erect, bends the legs slowly at the knees, and as he suddenly straightens them he simultaneously shoots his hand aloft. This motion will carry the bell to about level with the crown of the head, and then it loses its momentum. At that exact instant you must again bend the knees and squat under the bell, just as in Fig. 29. You will notice that this is exactly the position of one of the leg exercises. When a beginner starts to practice the "jerk," either with one hand or two hands, he is possessed with the idea that the first motion should carry the bell all the way to arms' length. So he will make a tremendous effort, which will carry the bell about 5 inches above the head, and then he will stand with the legs almost straight, and try to force the bell up the rest of the way by pure arm strength. You will probably do just that when you start to practice it, and if you do you must stop at once and learn the correct way. If you can master the second dip with the knees your record will be 50 to 100 lbs. better than if you attempt to force the bell up entirely by arm strength. The second dip with the knees is the most important part in the whole lift. Some lifters perform a sort of split in order to lower the body; that is, they spring forward with one foot and backward with the other.

Others step forward with one foot, and still others step backward with one foot. That is all lost motion. The correct thing is to drop the body straight downwards by sitting on the heels; which is the style used by Steinborn.

In making a right-arm jerk some lifters bend the body slightly to the left and allow the right arm to rest on the right side of the body, as in Fig. 68. In a two-arm jerk some lifters allow the handle bar to rest on the upper chest, as in Fig. 67, and jerk the bell off the body. Geo. Jowett holds the bell almost opposite his chin, and extends the elbows out to the front. That is an extremely scientific method, because before Jowett has started to raise the bell overhead, his elbows are half way up; whereas if a man holds his elbows down by his sides, as in Fig. 67, they have to travel twice as far as Jowett's do before the arms are straightened. But Mr. Jowett has a tremendous wrist and very thick forearms, and I doubt whether his style would be possible for everyone. However, it is interesting to know that Jowett at the weight of 158 lbs., and using his style, raised 286 lbs. in the two-arm jerk; whereas Steinborn, using the other style, raised 345 officially, and 375 unofficially, and Steinborn weighed 215 lbs. Since Jowett came closer than Steinborn to raising double his own weight, his style seems to be justified.

If you were reading a lifting-record book you would be very much confused by the multiplicity of records, unless you were posted regarding the styles used in different countries. In England and France the rules require that a lifter must raise the bell clean from the floor to shoulder before jerking it aloft. In fact, I believe that they still enforce that rule. The word "clean" signifies that the bell must be lifted in one motion to the chest without touching the body on its upward journey. In Germany and Austria the lifter was allowed to get the bell to the shoulders in any way that he pleased. If he were going to make a one-arm jerk he was permitted to take the bell in two hands and, with a mighty swing, bring it from the floor to in front of his right shoulder. Then he would let go with his left hand and make the jerk with the right arm. An English or French lifter would be disqualified if he did that. He was compelled to lift the bell with one hand all the way, and to use only his right arm in raising the bell to the shoulder, as well as in jerking it from the shoulder to overhead. In the two-arm jerk the French and English lifters raised the bell clean; but in Germany, Austria, and all the other European countries, the lifter could raise the bell from the floor, rest it on his abdomen, as in Fig. 71, then give a jump, get it across the lower part of his chest, and then with another jump get it opposite his neck and ready to jerk aloft. (Sometimes the rules were so lax that the lifter was allowed to wear a belt with a huge buckle in front. He would raise the bell and rest it on this buckle; then he would lean back from the waist and roll the bell up the front of his body. This is an easy trick for a stout man.) When you compare the foreign records you must take into consideration the method used. The French record is something like 345 lbs.; whereas, the Austrian record is almost 80 lbs. more. To the best of my knowledge and belief, the old record in the two-arm jerk, clean all the way, was Cyr's lift of 345 lbs. That record stood for years until Henry Steinborn, in Philadelphia, did 347¼ pounds under official conditions. Then, a week later, he did 375 lbs. unofficially. He thought he was lifting 350, but the men who loaded the bell made a miscalculation, and the bell actually weighed 375. Steinborn failed in his first two attempts, and got it up on his third attempt, because he knew in his heart and soul that he could do 350. When they weighed the bell and they found that he had done 375, he could hardly believe the news.

Before the War I used to subscribe to French, English and German magazines which were devoted to lifting and even then the German lifters sneered at the smallness of the French records, and the French in their turn, sneered at what they called "the

German's clumsy and unfair style." The only way in which I am interested in the controversy is in its relation to super strength.

CHAPTER XIII

ARM STRENGTH

Now we have finally gotten as far as your arms. If I had started out by telling you how to develop your upper-arm muscles, some of you would never have gone beyond that chapter, because the average physical culturist is firmly convinced that great strength depends entirely on the size and strength of the upper arms. Such arm exercises as have been given so far were incidental to the development of the shoulders and back. When you push barbells, dumbbells or kettle-bells aloft, as in Figs. 51, 52, and 53, you are doing the best possible exercise for developing the outer head of the triceps muscle. When you lift a kettle-bell, as in Fig. 49, you are developing the inner side of the arm, which is another part of the triceps muscle. To develop your biceps muscles, all you have to do is to take a bar-bell in your hands, palms forward, and slowly raise that bell by bending your arms at the elbows, until the bell is in position Fig. 72. The exercise will be easier if you keep your hands a little farther apart than the breadth of your shoulders. Another helpful thing is to bend the wrists and lift the palms of the hands before you start to bend the arms at the elbows. If you are small and light, 30 lbs. is enough to begin with; if you weigh 200 lbs. you can start with 60 or 65 lbs. After you can repeat the curling motion several times in succession without much exertion, add 5 or 10 pounds to the weight of the bell. After the weight has been increased you will be able to curl only two or three times; but after a few days' practice you can repeat as many times as you did with the lighter weight, and then you must make another weight increase and proceed as before.

When the bell is held with the palms in front, or what we call "the under-grip," the biceps muscle can exert more power than if you hold the palms down, (the overgrip). That is because the forearm muscles, which bring the palm towards the forearm, are stronger than the muscles which bring the back of the hand towards the forearm. If you have ever practiced chinning the bar, you have undoubtedly found that you can chin twice as often with the palms towards you as with the palms of the hands away from you. In curling a bar-bell you will raise anywhere from 50 to 75 per cent more by the under-grip than by the over-grip.

The biceps muscle, which bends the arm, is only about two-thirds as large and as strong as the triceps muscle, which straightens the arm. A well-developed man who can make a two-arm curl (under-grip) with 100 lbs., should be able to make a two-arm press with 140 or 150 lbs. (The two-arm press is nothing more nor less than the shoulder exercise illustrated in Fig. 51.) Curling a barbell with both hands, or a dumbbell with one hand, will give you big biceps muscles; but the curling should be used only as an exercise, and not as a feat of strength. In European competitions I have never known "curling" weights to be included in a program of competitive lifts; although it sometimes appears on the list of English lifts.

The biceps muscle is not nearly as important as you think it is. The amount of weight you can lift by a contraction of the biceps is paltry compared to the amount of weight you can lift by the strength of one leg, or by the contraction of even one of the muscles on your upper back. If you practice with a bar-bell you will be surprised to see how quickly you reach your limit in "curling" barbells. Your record in pressing a bar-bell to arms' length overhead will always be far better than your record in "curling" a bar-bell. Although I have seen many middle-sized men take a 200-lb. barbell in both hands and press it slowly to arms' length above the head, I have never yet seen a man perform a two-arm curl with a bell of that weight. I have seen lifters curl 100 lbs. with one arm, but they first placed the bell on the ground, and when they leaned over and took hold of the bell, they already had the arm slightly bent at the elbow, and as they straightened the legs it would give the bell a little bit of a start. The proper way to do a one-arm curl is to stand erect, with the bell in one hand and that arm hanging limp at the side. Then you can move the arm slightly forward, twist the bell so that your palm is front; and then, with the hand in the under-grip position, slowly bend the arm until you have lifted the bell to in front of the shoulder. While bending the arm, you should not lean back at the waist. Your body should be upright at all times. I have never seen 100 lbs. curled with one arm. There are, undoubtedly, men who can do this, but I have never happened to see one of them do it. I believe that Henry Steinborn, or either Joe or Adolph Nordquest could curl 100 lbs. with one hand, although I never heard any of them say that they have done so. I remember that Warren Travis once told me that he saw Horace Barre do a one-arm curl three times in succession, with a 100-lb. dumbbell. Furthermore, he said that Barre did not bother to rotate his arm and use the undergrip, but held the hand sideways, as in Fig. 73. If Barre had used the undergrip at the start of the curl, he would undoubtedly have curled 125 lbs. at least once; but then Barre weighed close to 300 lbs. himself, and it is not much of a trick to do a "one-arm curl" with a bell half your own weight. I saw Henry Steinborn do a two-arm curl five or six times in succession, with a bar-bell that weighed 173 lbs. (as in Fig. 130). It did not seem to be the least trouble to him. He was about to pose for some pictures, and he used the bar-bell for a few minutes to get his muscles flushed with blood so that they would be bigger and show up better in the photographs. Charles Herold, who weighed less than 160 lbs., could do a one-arm curl properly with 90 lbs., but when he curled 100 lbs. he would start the curl from the floor with his arm slightly bent. On one occasion Herold stood between two dumbbells, each of which weighed 103 lbs. He leaned over, curled one bell with the right hand in the style described, and then did a military press with the bell at arm's length above his head. He leaned over again, curled the other bell with his left hand, and slowly pushed it up alongside of the first bell. Each movement was either a slow curl or a slow military press.

In a recent article in Strength, Mr. Jowett made a statement that Louis Cyr once did a one-arm curl with a dumbbell weighing 238 lbs. I can believe most of the stories about Cyr, but with all due respect to Mr. Jowett, I can't believe that one. Cyr did a one-arm press with 273 lbs., and my friend, George Zottman, pressed 264 in almost exactly the same style that Cyr used. Zottman admits that he cannot do a correct one-arm curl with 100 lbs., and I doubt whether Cyr, who weighed 100 lbs. more than Zottman, could have done a one-arm curl with more than 165 lbs. at the outside.

(After I dictated the foregoing paragraphs, I went to see Zottman in order to get his opinion on the matter. He agreed with me in believing that it was impossible for Cyr to make a one- arm curl with 238 lbs. When I asked him his opinion as to whether Cyr could have "muscled-out" 135 lbs. with his right hand, he said that he could easily credit that feat, because he had, himself, once held out a 114-lb. dumbbell, although he was able to maintain it at arm's length for only one second. He first pressed the bell aloft and lowered it into position, and he showed me the position in which he stood. [It was something like Fig. 60, but he stood straighter and his right arm was not nearly so much bent; neither was his body bent as far to the left.] He said that he could muscle-out with one arm more than he could curl properly with one arm, and that he believes this is true of most "Strong Men" who can press big weights aloft with one arm. He further said that if he muscled-out 114 lbs., Cyr should certainly have muscled-out 135, because Cyr's arms were a little shorter and much thicker than his own.)

In a later chapter, I will show you how the size of the biceps is affected by the size of the forearm.

CHAPTER XIV

LIFTING A BAR-BELL FROM FLOOR TO CHEST

Now let us go back to the difference between the French and German styles of lifting. As I said before, when a German was going to make a one-arm jerk, he would lift the bell from the floor to the chest with both hands, and the Frenchman would lift it all the way with one hand.

If you ask a beginner to lift a heavy bar-bell with one hand to his shoulder, he will instinctively try to make the lift by arm-strength. He leans over, grasps the middle of the handlebar and slowly straightens up. This brings the bar-bell about opposite the middle of his thigh. Then he tries to get the weight still higher by bending the arm; that is, he tries to "curl" it. He quickly finds that his biceps' strength is not sufficient to raise the weight; so he leans his body back at the waist and tries to swing the bell outwards, and the only result is that the weight rises a few inches and then falls back against his thighs.

Here is the way a trained lifter manages it. The method is like that employed in the snatch, except that in the snatch you use the over-grip, but in lifting a bar-bell to the shoulder you use the under-grip. The lifter stoops down, as in Fig. 74, with his knees bent considerably, his body inclined forward from the hips and his back perfectly flat. His arm is as straight as a poker. He then "stands up" quickly; and if he puts enough vigor into the movement, and assists himself by pressing hard against the left knee with the left hand, the bell will fly up in the air until it is about opposite the nipples. Then the lifter bends his knees and lowers his body in a straight line, pulls the bell directly towards his shoulder; and from that point he can lift the bell aloft. If the bar-bell is a light one, a good lifter does not have to employ the second bend of the legs, because the first effort will be powerful enough to make the bell fly to shoulder-height. On the contrary, with a really heavy bell, the first movement will not bring the handlebar much higher than the waist-line; and then the lifter has to go into a deep crouch in order to pull the bell in towards his shoulder. (As in the overhand jerk, some lifters step backwards and some forwards. Some of them practically kneel on the knee of the right leg.)

When a dumbbell is used, it should be put fore and aft between the feet, and the lifter should start in the same way and swing the bell slightly outwards as he pulls it upwards; because it is necessary to turn the bell completely over to get it into pressing position. It is easier to lift a 150-lb. bar-bell clean to the shoulder than to do the same thing with a 120-lb. dumbbell.

In order to get a quick start for a 100-yard dash, the sprinter goes into a crouch, because it has been proven that a man can release more energy and get a quicker start in that position than if he stands upright. A football linesman, when about to charge his opponent, also goes into a crouch; he can push harder in that position. When a lifter is going to raise a heavy weight clean to the shoulder, he crouches almost as low as the sprinter does, although he does not bend either his back as far forward, or his legs quite as much at the knees.

There is another example of the superiority of bodily strength over arm strength. I have seen a man who could not make a correct one-arm curl with 75 lbs. pull a 200-lb. bar-bell clean to the shoulder with his right hand.

For some reason or other, when a French lifter pulls a bar-bell clean from floor to shoulder, he uses the over-grip, just as he does in the snatch; and just why the French should elect to handicap themselves in this way, is hard to decide. In May, 1917, at an exhibition in my factory, Anton Matysek tried to make a record for himself in the one-arm clean and press; but for some reason he used the over-grip in pulling the bell from floor to shoulder. He did 190 lbs. easily and failed at 201. I told him then, and I am still convinced, that if he had used the under-grip he could have pulled 220 lbs. to the shoulder quite easily. The palm of his hand would have been toward him when the bell was at the shoulder, and in order to get the bell in position for the press, all that would have been necessary was to swing the right hand end of the bell backwards. By using the over-grip he landed himself in position, Fig. 75; and then, in order to get the bell so that he could press it, he had to swing the left hand end backwards and duck far to the left, so that the handlebar could pass over his head. However, that position has nothing to do with the fact that he deliberately restricted the amount he could lift to his shoulder through using the over-grip. At that time he could press aloft from the shoulder 240 lbs., any time he tried to do so, and occasionally he'd go over 250 lbs. Therefore, if he had started by using the under-grip, he would have made a record of at least 220, "clean" all the way. As it was, he didn't even get a chance to try to press 201, because he failed—through using the over-grip—to bring the weight to his shoulder.

There is a French, or French-Swiss, family called De Riaz; and three brothers of that name, Emile, George and Maurice, are among the most famous of European lifters. Any one of them

126

can do 180 lbs. in a one-arm swing and 190 lbs. in a one-arm snatch. I think it was Emile who made a one-arm swing with 193¼, and Maurice who did a one-arm clean and jerk with 231 lbs. George Lurich, who in his youth was one of the world's greatest lifters, lifted from the floor to the shoulder, with two hands, and then jerked aloft with the right arm, a bar-bell weighing 266½ lbs. From what I have seen of Henry Steinborn, I am sure that he could break either of these records with ease. He once promised me that if there was sufficient inducement, he would make a one-arm jerk with 270 lbs., clean all the way, and a one- arm jerk of 300 lbs., two hands to the shoulder.

Arthur Saxon, whose best public record in the one-arm snatch was around 200 lbs., could pull a 300-lb. bar-bell "clean" to the shoulder, and then "bent-press" it to arms' length. Anything that Saxon could do in the "clean lifts" or the "quick lifts," Steinborn can beat by five percent.

Lifting a bell to the shoulder with two hands, preparatory to a one-hand overhead lift, is a comparatively simple matter. You grasp the middle of the bar with the right hand, under-grip, and with your left hand you take an over-grip, the fingers of the left hand encircling the knuckles of the right hand. From the half-crouch, you straighten up and lift with both arms. In some countries it is allowed to stand a bar-bell on end and rock it into position, but that is more a matter of leverage than strength. Fig. 76 shows Matysek about to rock a 220-lb. bell to the shoulder. First, he will tilt the bell until the upper sphere is away from him; then he will make the bell lean in the other direction, so that the upper sphere will fall over his shoulder. As he does this, he will slide the palm of his left hand down the underside of the handle and toward the lower sphere. When the top end of the bell commences to dip backwards, he will allow his legs to bend at the knees, and with his left hand he will raise the front sphere;

which will make the bell slowly topple into a horizontal position. Then he will stand erect by straightening the legs and be in a position to start his press.

In lifting a bar-bell with two hands clean to the shoulder, you use the over-grip. When you straighten the body from the crouch, the bell flies up to opposite your chest, and the elbows will be pointed outward and upwards. Then, when the bell loses its momentum, you have to bring your elbows down like a flash and at the same time pull the bell towards you; and if you do the movement correctly, your forearms will be vertical under the handlebar and your upper arms pressed against the sides of your chest; and just as in the other clean lifts, some lifters step forward, some backward, and the best ones squat straight down. The French authorities used to claim that the world's record in the two-arm clean and jerk was Arvid Anderson's 328 lbs., although Des Bonnet recognized Cyr's 345 lbs. Steinborn's official 347½ is the present record, and his unofficial 375 lbs. has never been approached. In German and Austrian competitions the rules formerly required (and may still require) that a lifter about to make a two-arm press should raise the bell clean to the chest; as it was considered that anyone should be able to raise clean to the chest the amount of weight which he could press to arms' length; because in the press you use the strength of the arms and the shoulders, without any assistance from the legs. As said in Chapter 12, the lifter about to make a two-arm jerk, was allowed to raise the weight to the chest in any way he pleased. I have no partiality for the Germans and Austrians, but in any discussion of weight-lifting, it is necessary to take those nations into account, because they numbered their lifters by the tens of thousands. The reason that they had a number of men who could raise over 370 lbs. in the two-arm jerk, while France had none who could raise 350, and England none who could raise 325, was because the German rules permitted the lifters to practice with heavier weights. For a long time the French and English lifters never had a chance to show what they really could do in a two-arm jerk, because the amount of weight they could handle in that lift was limited by the amount they could raise clean to the chest. I am not interested in any controversy between the German- Austrian lifters on the one hand and the French-English lifters on the other, but I am vitally interested in knowing the amount of weight which can be lifted by the strength of any muscle or set of muscles. Since everyone knows that a lifter can raise from his shoulders to arms' length above the head a greater weight than he can bring clean from the floor to the chest, it is perfectly plain that any lifter, whatever his nationality, who restricts himself to the "clean" style will never be able to reach the limit of his powers in the overhead lift. For several years the world's record in the two-arm jerk was held by William Tuerk, an Austrian giant, who lifted 364 lbs., and the citizens of Vienna were so proud of him that they presented him with the freedom of the city. His record was later eclipsed by several other Austrians, Tandler, Grafl, Eicheldrat, Witzelsberger and Steinbach. Steinbach took a 386-lb. bar-bell to the shoulders and jerked it aloft twice in succession. About 1912 a new star appeared in the person of Karl Swaboba. This man, while not very tall, was immensely broad and weighed about 320 lbs. (He should not be confused with the Mr. Swoboda who is prominent in physical culture circles in this country.) I understand that Swaboba of Vienna made a two-arm press with 352 lbs., and a two-arm jerk with 402 lbs.; and that in that latter lift it took him five separate motions to raise the bell from the floor to the chest. When he did get it to his chest, he jerked it aloft quite easily. It is further said that on one occasion he made a two-arm jerk with 440 lbs. after four men had lifted the bell to his chest. I do not guarantee the accuracy of the foregoing figures, because I have lost, or given away, most of my old books and magazines which dealt with the subject.

This is not a book about records, nor does it pretend to tell you all about the most scientific methods of performing the standard lifts. One could write a book of considerable size, and deal with nothing except records and the way they were made. What we are concerned with is the creation of bodily strength; and since bodily strength is a great factor in the two-arm jerk, I have to devote a good deal of time to that lift. If you are going to practice it, I certainly advise you to learn the so-called "continental" method of raising the bell to the chest, for otherwise you will be unable to determine how much you really can raise in a two- arm jerk.

Authorities on scientific lifting claim that a well-trained and very skillful man, who has great agility as well as great bodily strength, should be able to raise, in a two-arm jerk, fifty percent more than he can raise in the two-arm press. This is a most inter- esting subject, because investigation proves that a middle-sized man, well developed and quick in his movements, can deliver much more power in proportion to his bodily weight than can the big giants. Cyr could make a two-arm press with 315 lbs., and could do only about ten per cent more if he used the jerk. When Swaboba did all the lifting himself, his best record in the jerk was less than fifteen percent better than his best record in the press. Arthur Saxon, who weighed about 200 lbs., and was exceedingly quick for a big man, showed a difference of about thirty-three and a third percent, as his records were 260 in the press and 345 in the jerk. Steinborn, who was the quickest heavy man I have ever seen, showed a difference of about forty percent for he has raised 375 in the two-arm jerk clean all the way, and I believe that his best record in the press is about 265.

There are a number of men weighing around 140 to 150 lbs. who have reached the fifty-percent standard. Max Sick, who weighed about 145 lbs., succeeded in raising 330 lbs. in the two- arm jerk, and I understand that his best record in the two-arm press was about 220 lbs. There are several of the European lifters in the 140 to 150-lb. class who can make a two-arm press with about 200 lbs. and a two-arm jerk with about 300 lbs. The ambition of every lifter is to raise double his own weight aloft in the two-arm jerk. So far there are less than a dozen men who have done this, and they are comparatively small men. I know two or three amateurs in this country who are rapidly approaching that standard. This matter of the two-arm jerk should be a great source of satisfaction to the lifter of average size, because it proves that a man does not necessarily have to be a giant in size or weight in order to be possessed of super-strength. Just think! little Max Sick, weighing 143 pounds, did 330 in a two-arm jerk; and the gigantic Swaboda, who weighed over 300 (which is twice as much as Sick weighed), could raise only about 70 lbs. more than the smaller man could.

Super-strength is as much a matter of muscular development and co-ordination as it is of mere size and bulk. The middle-sized man who can raise twice his weight in the two-arm jerk is a far better athlete than the giant who can raise only a little more than his own weight. Moreover, super-strength positively can be cultivated, which is a very satisfying thought.

In the old days of lifting, that is, up to forty years ago, American athletes were acquainted with only one style of pushing a weight overhead. At that time such a thing as a bar-bell was almost unknown, although there were plenty of short-handled dumbbells. The best lifter of those days was the man who could take the heaviest dumbbell in his right hand, swing it to his shoulder, and then, while standing erect, push it slowly to arm's length overhead. In weight-lifting circles that is known as a one-arm "military" press. The lifter is required to stand with the heels together, the legs straight and, as the name implies, to keep his body as upright as that of a soldier standing "at attention." In some parts of the world the lifter is made to stand with the left hand pressed against the outside of his left thigh, and in other parts he is allowed to hold the left arm horizontally to the side. The lift to the shoulder is unimportant, because the weight used is not very heavy; but after it is at the shoulder, you have to hold the bell slightly away from you and slightly in front of you, as in Fig. 78, and then slowly push it up; and if you lean your shoulders back an inch, or an inch to the left, you're disqualified. The force which lifts the bell is supplied by a contraction of the deltoid muscle on the point of the right shoulder and the triceps muscle on the back of the arm. The body muscles are involved because they have to keep the body in an upright position; the legs have but little to do. It is much harder to bring your arm directly overhead when the body is held erect than when you lean the body over sideways or forwards; because when you do lean the body over you are pushing the arm more out to the side, even though the bell travels up in a vertical line.

Arthur Saxon, who could make a one-arm bent press with 336 lbs., could not military-press 130 lbs.; and Sandow, who had a bent-press record of 271, could military-press only 121. The "military press" is a test of pure arm and shoulder strength, and, as I will show you in a later chapter, the bent-press is a feat of bodily strength. I can't tell you the record in the military press. In a previous book I said that Witzelsberger, of Vienna, had done 154 lbs., but I have since been told that while Witzelsberger kept his heels together and his legs straight, he bent his body over slightly. It is said that Cyr once made a military press with a 165-lb. bar-bell, and Mr. Jowett says he saw the giant, La Vallee, do 165 lbs. The tradition is that Michael Meyer could make a one-arm military press of 150 pounds without much trouble. (This is the same man who is said to have muscled-out 112 lbs. to the front.) When doing a "Strong" act with a circus, Meyer would stand with his back to one of the tent-poles. Attendants would wind a rope around his body, binding it fast to the post, but leaving his right arm free. He would hold his right hand in front of the right shoulder, and the attendants would put a 150-lb. bell in it, and Meyer would slowly push it aloft. This is not as hard as it sounds, because the ropes which encircled Meyer's body gave him a splendid brace. The man who can make the biggest one-arm military press is the man who can muscle-out the heaviest weight; which proves that a powerful shoulder muscle is the thing that counts most. The fact that Cyr could military-press 165 lbs is explained by his ability to muscle-out 135 lbs.; and the same thing applies to Meyer, to Zottman and others of the big men.

Last summer I saw Robert Snyder make a beautiful one-arm military press with 91 lbs., and he weighed only a little over 140 lbs. He just failed in 96 lbs. He put the bell up easily enough, but he bent a little bit to the side.

In a two-arm military press, the weight should be lifted clean and then pressed aloft without any backward bend of the body or without the slightest bend of the legs. Your record in the two-arm military press should be nearly double your record in the one- arm military press. Shoulder strength is just as important, and back strength is also necessary. If you are of average size, the bell you would use in a one-arm military press is not as heavy as you are, probably not half as heavy as you are; but in a two-arm press it is possible to use more than your own weight, and in order to keep the body upright, your back must be very strong. The reason I can believe that Cyr made a one-arm military press with 165 lbs. is because his record in the two-arm press is 315, and they say that he hardly leaned back at all when he made that two-arm press.

"Military-pressing," like "muscling-out," is a test of strength rather than an exercise. In making a regular two-arm press, the athlete is allowed to stand with the feet apart and one foot slightly in advance; but he must not bend the legs after the weight has been brought to the chest or while he is pushing it aloft; although he is allowed to lean considerably backwards from the waist.

There is an intermediate lift between the two-arm press and the two-arm jerk that is sometimes called "the push." After the bell is at the chest, the lifter leans his shoulders forward and brings his hips backwards, as in Fig. 79; and then, as he suddenly pushes the bell aloft, he brings his hips forward and bends over backward, as in Fig. 80. I can see no particular advantage in this style of lifting, either as a competitive event or as a training exercise. You can raise more by the "push" than by the press, but not so much as by the jerk. In one-arm lifting, you accomplish a right-arm push by standing with the feet apart and then bending to the right, as in Fig. 81; and then swinging the body to the left and slightly forward as you push the bell aloft, as in Fig. 82. A very strong workman or athlete seems to instinctively adopt this style the first time he tries to "push up" a heavy dumbbell.

There is also a variation called "the side press," and that can be dealt with in another chapter.

PLATE 39

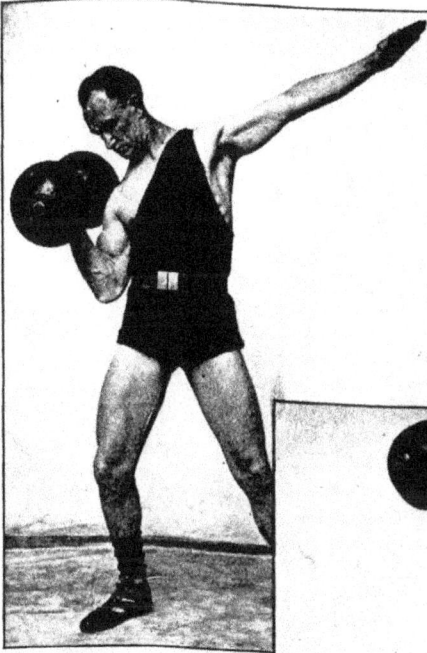

Fig. 81

Plate 39, Figure 81 (above), showing the start of the one-arm "Push." The lifter stands with the feet well apart, leans to the right, and rests most of his weight on the right leg

Fig. 82

Then he shifts his weight to the left leg, swings his body sharply to the left, and pushes the bell aloft by a mighty thrust of his arm, as in Figure 82 (below). It is possible to lift almost twice as much in this style as in a "Military Press," but not nearly as much can be raised in a one-arm "Push" as by a one-arm "Bent Press," a lift which is described later in the book

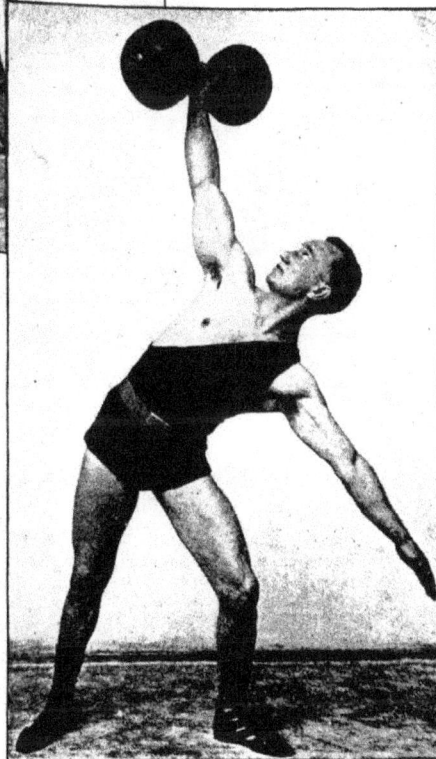

PLATE 40

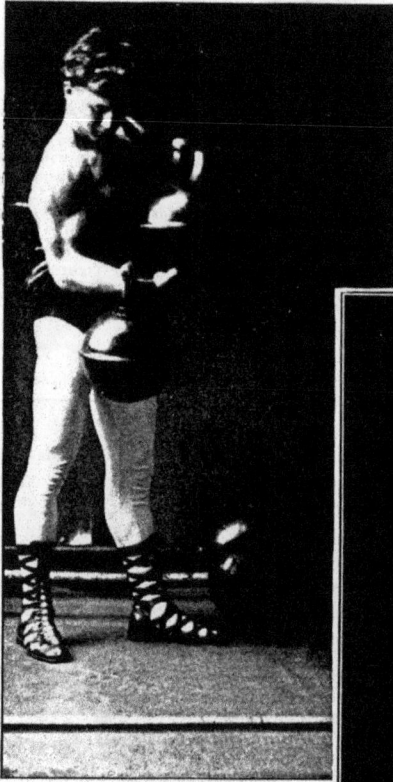

Fig. 83

Plate 40, Figure 83 (above).
F. R. Rohde, a young Western athlete, with a magnifi-
c e n t development. H i s
thighs are extraordinarily
large in proportion to his
hips and waist. (See text.)

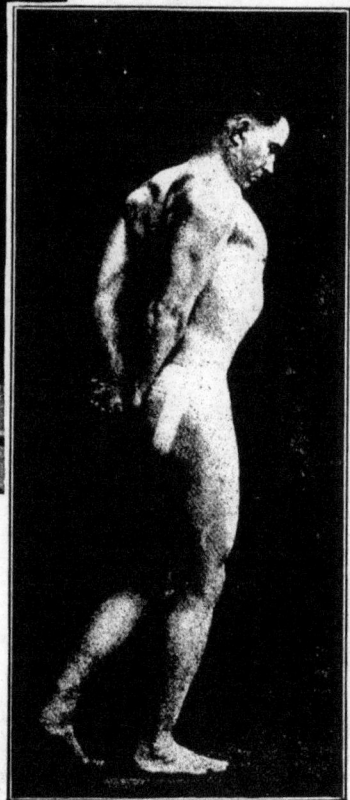

Fig. 84

Figure 84 (below). Frank
Dilks, who started to train at
the age of twenty-eight, who
increased his chest measurement nine inches in one year,
and whose hips gained at
least five inches in girth

PLATE 41

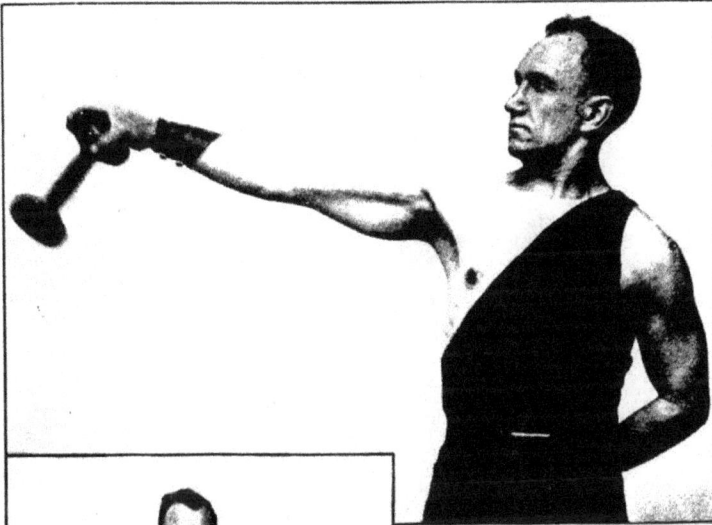

Fig. 85

Plate 41, Figure 85 (above)
A good exercise to develop
the muscles of the hand and
the forearm. One end of the
dumbbell must be rested in
the palm of the hand, and
gripped by the finger-tips.
The free end of the dumb
bell is waved around in
circles, first forward, and
then backward.

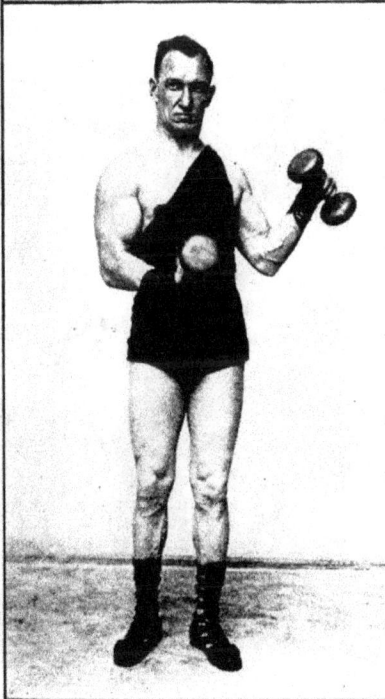

Fig. 86

Figure 86 (below). The Zott
man exercise, which is un
equaled for developing the
forearms.

PLATE 42

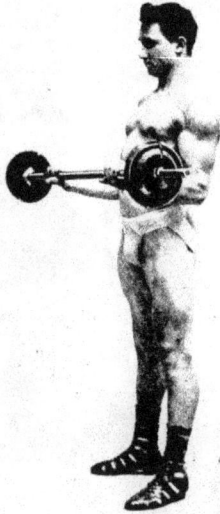

Fig. 87

Plate 42, Figure
(above). Curling
light bar-bell with th
"over grip"—that i
knuckles up, to d
velop the muscles o
the outsides of th
forearm

Fig. 88

Figure 88 (below). Matysek
curling with the over grip
a bar-bell with a handle
nearly three inches thick.
For a description of this particular feat, read the chapter
on forearm exercises

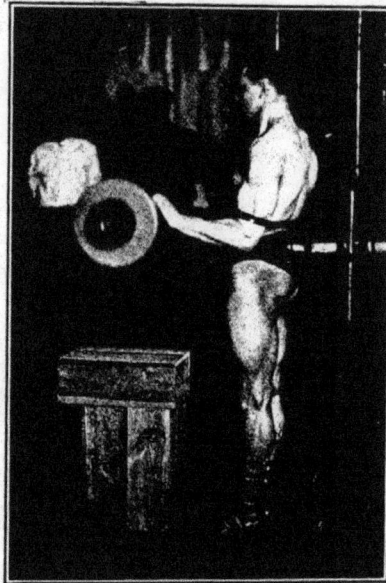

PLATE 43

Fig. 89

Plate 43 Figure 89 (above), showing how to lift with one finger at a time in order to increase the strength of the fingers. Several successive lifts with 75 or 100 lbs. will develop more finger strength than one lift with a heavier weight. You can lift with the first finger alone, or the middle finger alone, but the third and little fingers should always be used together.

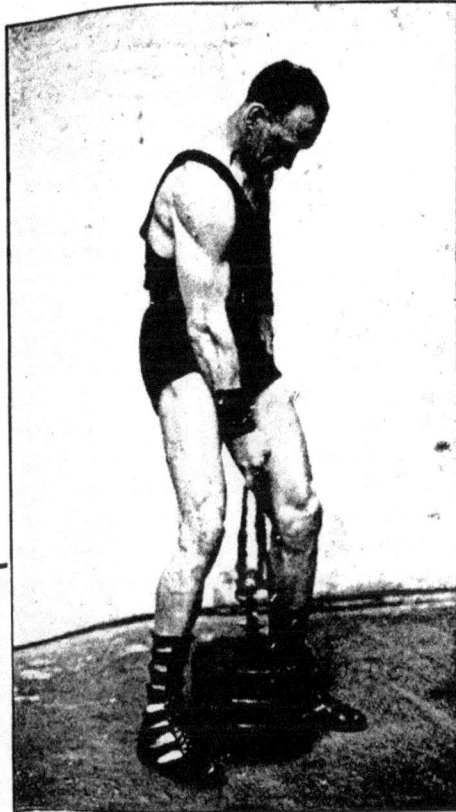

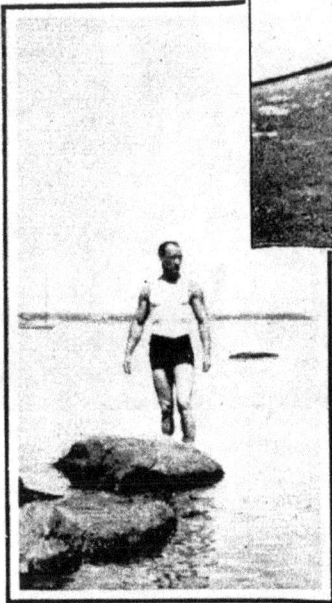

Fig. 90

Figure 90 (below). A snapshot of Walter Donald in beach costume. Mr. Donald kindly volunteered to pose for many of the exercise pictures in this book. You can identify him by his magnificent arm development.

PLATE 44

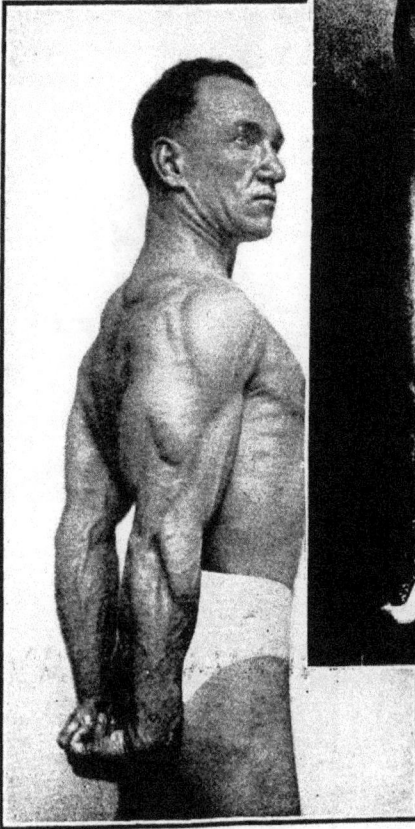

Fig. 91

Plate 44, Figure 91
(above). Robert Snyder
posing with the elbow
raised so as to contract
the biceps muscle to its
fullest extent

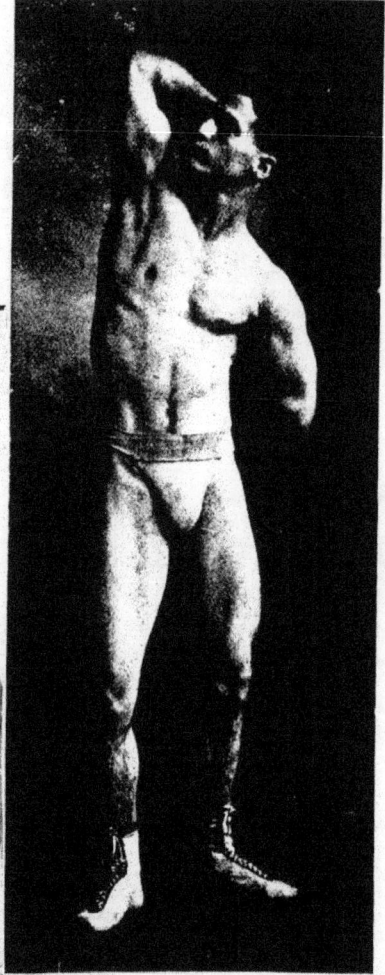

Fig. 92

Figure 92 (below). Walter
Donald with his arms placed
so as to show the triceps
muscles to the greatest advantage

PLATE 45

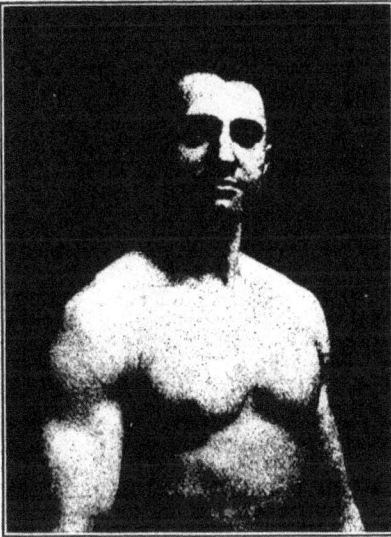

Fig. 93

Plate 45, Figure 93
(above). Anton Mat-
ysek with all his mus-
cles relaxed, showing
breast m u s c l e s so
highly developed that
they sag slightly of
their own weight

Fig. 94

Figure 94 (below).
Showing the difference
in the shape of the
chest, arm, and shoul-
der muscles after Mat-
ysek has flexed them
by mental control

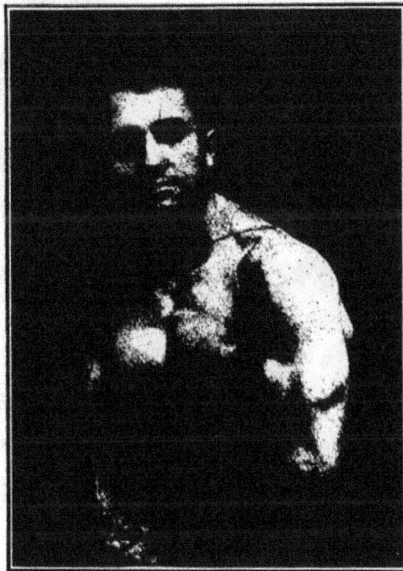

141

PLATE 46

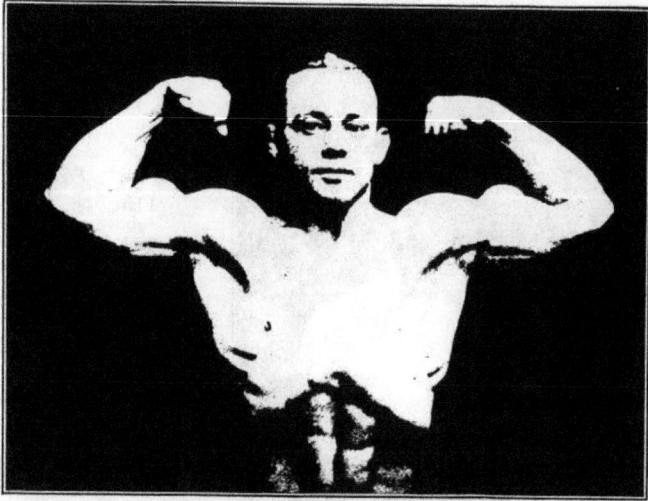

Fig. 95

Plate 46, Figure 95 (above). Otto Arco, who weighs 145 lbs., and who is one of the best lifters of his size in the world. He learned "muscle control" after he had developed himself by lifting bar-bells

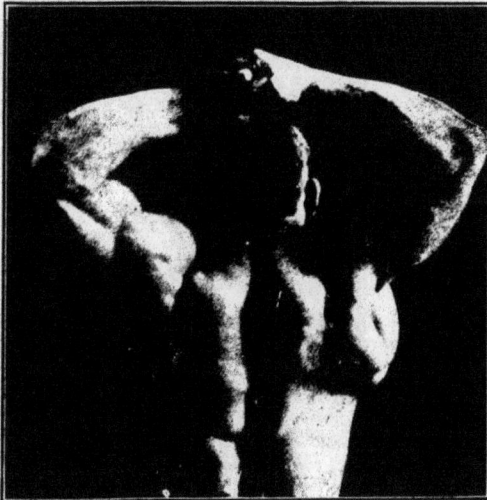

Fig. 96

Figure 95 shows the "Rope" or isolated control of the abdominal muscles. Figure 96 (below), shows his ability to control his shoulder blades

CHAPTER XV

ON INDIVIDUAL TRAINING

Besides the lifts described in the preceding chapters, there are two or three dozen others which are recognized in different countries; for example, the British Amateur Weight Lifting Association lists 47 distinct lifts, all of which are considered standard lifts. To describe them all would take a lot of space; and while it would add to your knowledge of lifting, it would not teach you much about developing yourself.

If you could read my daily mail, you would soon come to agree with me that the general public is far more interested in finely-developed bodies than in weight-lifting records. When Sandow toured America, the people flocked to see him. If 3000 men attended one of his performances, it is safe to say that not 300 of them could the next day have told you how many pounds Sandow had lifted; but each and every one of the 3000 would probably have told you that Sandow was the finest physical specimen he had ever seen. For every one man who says, "I would like to lift as much as Sandow did," there are one hundred men who will say, "I wish I could get a build like Sandow's." There was a time when I thought that lifting-records were the only thing that counted; whereas, I now think that records are comparatively unimportant, and that the development of the individual is all important. If I get a written report from a student of bar-bell work, the first things I want to know are whether his chest is getting bigger, his arms and legs assuming a certain size and shape, and what he weighs. His lifts are of minor importance, especially if he, like most pupils, is using the bar-bells for the sake of getting a better build and more muscular and organic vigor. In England, a man who uses a bar-bell seems to think of nothing except the amount of weight he can lift. Consequently, he devotes his entire practice time to mastering the niceties of the lifting game. In this country, the vast majority of bar-bell users have but little use for lifting records and are after bodily improvement first, last and all the time, which is just as it should be.

Within the last year, I have received hundreds of letters in which the writer would finish by saying, "I am convinced that by using adjustable bar-bells I can make myself much bigger and stronger and healthier; but I have no desire to become a professional lifter or to ever publicly exhibit my strength. If I use a bar-bell, is it necessary for me to do the muscle-racking stunts that I have seen on the professional stage, and will I be compelled to use tremendously heavy weights?" (The wording of the different letters may vary a bit; but the foregoing is the way the average letter reads.) Invariably, I tell the writers of those letters that a man who uses a bar-bell does not have to do any sensational lifting stunts in order to become either beautifully proportioned, very strong, or very healthy. Many of the writers of such letters are middle-aged men; and why should a man of forty try to become a record-breaking lifter? If I answer such letters, I say that if I can take a man and lay out for him a course of progressive exercises, which will give him a better shape and far more physical and vital energy than he had when he was twenty-one, then I do not care a particle about how many pounds he can lift.

Now understand, I like to watch a lifting contest, especially if the competitors are well-trained and highly-skilled lifters. Although I have seen a great deal of informal lifting and impromptu contests, it has been twenty years since I have been able to seat myself in the audience and watch a big public exhibition or competition. If I were present at such an affair, it was because I had gotten up the program and had to act as announcer, master of ceremonies and special reporter; and so,

144

at the end of the affair, I was much more tired than any of the competitors were.

I still like to see a first-class man make a big lift. I quite naturally feel elated if I see a friend, or a pupil, create a new record; but even then, I do not get the same solid satisfaction as I do when some other man writes a letter to tell me, that by practicing developing exercises with a bar-bell, he has restored himself to complete health; or that he has, by several months' steady practice, converted himself from a thin, undeveloped chap into an athlete of the Sandow-Matysek-Carr type. In the case of boys and very young men, one gets used to hearing of cases like that and one gets to take it as a matter of course; but when you get such a report from a man who was thirty-five or forty years old when he started to train, you get a feeling that you have witnessed a miracle. I have seen so many "near-miracles" accomplished through training with bar-bells, that I sometimes wonder why people waste time on other training methods.

Right here I want to interject a bit of caution. If you ever buy a bar-bell, the chances are nine out of ten, that you will become fascinated with the lifting end of the game; especially with lifting bar-bells or dumbbells to arms' length overhead. If you do that, you will deliberately interfere with your own progress to such an extent that you will never get as big or as strong as it is possible for you to be. When a man starts training with a bar-bell, the sensible thing to do is to adjust the bell to moderate weights; and, in each exercise, the weight of the bell should be adjusted to suit the strength of the muscle, or set of muscles, which are used in that exercise. Since some muscles are much bigger and vastly stronger than other muscles, it is naturally impossible to develop all the muscles to the limit by using a bar-bell of one fixed weight. For a beginner, even a 50-lb. bar-bell would be too heavy for use in some of the single-arm and shoulder exercises, although it might be too light to be used in such exercises as those described in Chapters 2 and 4.

The first thing to do is to increase the size of the chest, and to increase the strength of the lower back, and the size and strength of the thighs. During the first two months' practice, the arm and shoulder exercises are comparatively unimportant. Notwithstanding this, an uninstructed beginner usually spends almost all his time trying to develop his upper arm by pushing heavy weights aloft. When you start training, you must keep a tight rein on yourself; otherwise, you will plunge right into overhead lifting. The darned thing is so fascinating that there is a temptation to continually "try yourself out" to see whether you can push up a pound or two more than you did the day before. Then some friend drops in and says, "Bill, I hear you're training with a bar-bell. How much can you put up with one hand?" Such is your pride that you immediately proceed to "show" him. Then HE wants to try it; and if he has never seen any other bar-bell than yours, the chances are that he won't lift nearly as much as you can, even if you have been training for only two or three weeks. So he goes out and hunts up some big husky friend that he thinks can beat you, and brings that fellow around. The first thing you know,- instead of practicing your developing exercises in private, your exercise hour becomes a sort of reception, and all the time is spent in trying to outdo your visitors.

All the training during the first few months should be done in the privacy of your own room, or your own cellar. You can use a bar-bell in any space where you can use a pair of 5-lb. dumbbells. When practicing actual lifting, it is sometimes necessary to let the bell fall; although I know men who have become star lifters by practicing in their own rooms, and they never dropped a bell. In practicing the developing exercises, there is no likelihood nor necessity, for dropping a bell.

The reason for privacy is the necessity for intense concentration on the work. I do not mean that you have to grit your teeth and get red in the face, or flex your muscles by mental effort; but that you do have to pay a lot of attention to the way you are doing the different exercises. In any exercise, a few repetitions performed correctly are of more benefit than three times as many repetitions performed in a slovenly manner. If you feel that you must invite someone to watch you practice, pick out some chap who is familiar with bar-bell work and who will be able to explain to you the details of the exercises. After you have gotten your strength and development, then, if you want to practice lifting, you can take your bar-bell to a gymnasium; but you should pick out a gymnasium that is patronized by other lifting enthusiasts. By that time you will have gotten a very good idea of the measure of your own powers, and you will know just how much you can lift; and when you lean over and lift a bell from the floor, you will be able to make a very accurate estimate of its weight, and can tell by instinct whether or not it is in your power to lift it in a certain manner. Since the other lifters will have just the same experience and the same good judgment, the lot of you can practice competitive lifting and learn a good deal by studying the lifting style of the various members of the group.

If you suggest to the average undeveloped man that he take up bar-bell exercises as mean of development, he will reply, "Oh, I don't want that kind of exercise! It's too much like work. All my friends go to a gym, and play handball, or join the class- drills." The proper answer would be, "Well, what do your friends look like after they have spent two or three years at class- drills?"

Class-work is a lot of fun. You meet your friends; and after a lot of dilly-dallying, you stand up in rows and try to imitate the different movements of the instructor. You stretch your muscles, shake up your liver, get in a mild perspiration and give your lungs a little moderate work. When the drill is over, you all troop to the showers and do a lot of shouting; and afterwards, you all go away telling each other how "perfectly bully" you feel. After the first two or three sessions, any excuse is good enough to keep from going to the next class-drill. If you did keep it up all winter, you'd be benefited to some extent. Your muscles would work easier and would gain in tone. Your digestion would probably improve, and so would your complexion. Understand me, almost any kind of exercise is good; but class-drills are more like play than serious work. When an instructor is about to give a drill to a large group of men, he has to gauge the severity of the work by the capability of the average member. Therefore, if you are bigger and stronger and more athletic than the average, you feel that you're being kept at kindergarten stunts; and if you happen to be fat, middle-aged and out of condition, you feel that you're holding back the progress of the rest of the class. In many gyms there are what is known as "leaders' classes"; but I believe that such classes devote themselves, not to body-building work, but to the performance of elaborate stunts on the rings, the vaulting- horse or horizontal-bar exercises.

I have always been very much more interested in individual supremacy than in mass results. A regiment of soldiers drilling, or a couple of hundred gymnasts performing a mass-drill, bore me exceedingly. The very fact that so many individuals are doing the same thing, or making the same movements, is the best possible proof that those movements are easy to perform. If I go to a performance of an opera, I endure the singing of the chorus until the principals are again on the stage. You would have to pay me to make me sit through a performance of an oratorio, or a cantata, by a big chorus; although I would pay a high price to hear an individual singing star, like Ruffo or Chaliapin, Hempel or Destinn. If I go to the Russian Ballet, I feel that that part of the time is wasted when I have to watch forty or fifty girls doing toe-dancing movements or other evolutions at the same time; but when a great star like Nijinsky, or Nordkoff, or Pavlowa dances, I am all eyes, and I feel that I am getting more than my money's worth.

When it comes to gymnastics and athletics or body-building work, I carry my likes and dislikes even further. One time there was a big convention of gymnasts, and the main feature was a mass-drill by 1000 men, who came from gymnasiums all over the country. I was specially invited; and the men who promoted the affair never could understand why I did not go to the Exhibition. The reason was that on the same night I had chance to see at a local theatre, the performance of a pair of wonderful hand-balancers. Both of these men were superbly developed and enormously strong. They were living examples of what can be accomplished by specialized and individualized training. In order to do their act, each one of them had to have far more strength, agility and suppleness, than is possessed by the average athlete; and I learned more and got more satisfaction by watching them, than I could possibly have gotten by watching 1000 average gymnasts of average strength do average stunts.

Therefore, I am not very much impressed if I read a report stating that a class of forty men spent a winter at gymnastic training, and that at the end of the season, the average gain was I inch in chest measurement, inch in arm measurement, inch in leg measurement, and 5 lbs. in weight; because I know that the weakest member of that class, if trained individually, could have grained 4, or maybe 6, inches around the chest; 2 inches around the arms, and 3 inches around the thighs; and gained 15 to 25 lbs. in bodily weight. You can't get results like that in class work. Moderate improvement can be made by class work; but great improvement is a matter of individual instruction, individual training and individual study. It is just as impossible for the best instructor in body-building to give individual instruction to a class of twenty-four, as it would be for a great music teacher to give twenty-four pupils real results if he made them sit down at twenty-four pianos and play the same music at the same time. If a gymnastic instructor could take twenty-four pupils one at a time and give each one of them fifteen or thirty minutes' special instruction, he could perform wonders with the majority of them; but that would not be class teaching, but individual teaching.

There is no "simple and easy" way of getting a magnificently built body and the super-strength which goes with such development. It is just the same as in any other work that you do for the purpose of improving yourself. In the columns of some magazines, you will find advertisements which claim that if you pay a fee of $2.00 or $3.00, you will be sent a "new method" which will convert you into a first-class pianist in the few weeks it takes to complete that special course of lessons. There must be people who believe such statements, because the advertisements continue to appear; yet if you know anything at all about music, you also know that it takes several years' study before a pianist reaches the front rank of players. If you went to a good music teacher and told him that you wanted to become a piano player like Paderewski or Hoffman or Godowsky, he would reply, "Well, I will teach you all that I can; and you will have to give up a lot of time to it and practice several hours a day. After I am through with you, you may have to go abroad for a year or two and work in one of the big conservatories, or go to a man like Letzitsky for special coaching." If you did make such progress that a trip to Europe was justified, you would go with the foreknowledge that you would have to work and study even harder under the great coach, then under the preliminary coach; and that the large sums of money you would have to pay would not be for drills in the elementary part of the work, but for special knowledge. To get a magnificently developed body is a much easier matter than to become a great musician; but the principle is the same. You will never get to be very strong by elementary gymnastic exercises, any more than you will get to be a great pianist by practicing easy five-finger exercises for a few months. To master the piano or any other instrument, the performer has to learn the theory of music as well as the technical mastery of the keyboard. If a man of average size, poor health and little development, wishes to get the strength, shape and physical energy of a Sandow, it is not sufficient to know just which exercises to do. He must know how to do them, and why he does them.

A knowledge of muscular anatomy is a great help to anyone who is taking a body-building course. There are over 200 muscles in the body; and at first glance, it seems as though it would be a tremendous task to learn the names of those 200 muscles, where they are, what they do, and how to develop them. If you are interested, the knowledge will come easily. I know men who can instantly tell you the 1923 batting average of any of the 200 baseball players in the big leagues. They carry those figures, and a lot of other baseball dope, in their heads. They did not study hard to get that information, but absorbed it in the course of their daily reading of the sporting pages. If you use your muscles intelligently, it won't be more than a few days before you know the names of the principal muscles and what they do; and it will not be much longer before you know the names of practically all the muscles. Such knowledge of anatomy is not absolutely necessary; but it is a great help.

CHAPTER XVI

MAKING YOURSELF OVER

Of course you spend some of your time in reading books and stories. Every once in a while you read a book where the hero, who is of average build, disappears from the scene for some reason or other; and when he reappears, after an absence of a couple of years, his friends fail to recognize him. When they are convinced that he is the same man, they say, "But what has happened to you? You are about 4 inches wider and about 8 inches more around the chest than you used to be." In the last three months, I have read two such books. In one of them, the hero's family got into some financial difficulty, and he got a job on a fishing boat in the North Sea; and in the space of two years, he raised himself from seaman to mate. In the other story, the hero was supposed to be threatened with consumption and was sent away to a logging camp in our own Northwest; and when he returned, had affected a complete physical transformation.

These story-writers might be suspected of using a scene like that so that their heroes could have a fine shape and the. great strength that every well-regulated hero should have; but at that, they are not very far from the truth. I have known such things to happen in certain cases. I knew a man who went to the Klondike in the first gold rush. When he left this city, he was 23 years old and weighed, maybe, 135 lbs. When he returned two years later, he was no taller; but he weighed 185 lbs., and he did not carry an ounce of surplus flesh. He seemed to be all bone and muscle. On his outward journey, he wore a size 36 coat, which hung loosely on his shoulders. On his return journey, he wore a size 42 coat, which fitted him closely. His shoulders were very much broader; his arms and legs thicker; and even his wrist and ankles were bigger. Also, I have known other men who went away for a couple of years and lived in the outdoors, and came back no bigger than they were when they started. It happened that the first man had done a whole lot of hard work, had climbed mountains, dug ditches, paddled canoes and carried heavy packs over long trails. Of course the pure air and the outdoor life helped him; but pure outdoor air is not enough in itself to account for such an enormous increase in size and strength.

If the heroes in those two novels made the gains which the authors claim, it means that those two particular heroes did a lot of hard muscular work. I understand that in a lumber camp, the work is very hard, and it involves the lifting, handling and moving of very heavy weights. It takes more than a little muscle to swing an axe, and to cut down a tree which is a couple of feet thick. It takes even more muscle to stand at one end of a two-man saw, and saw that tree into sections. The peavey, or "cant-hook," which lumbermen use in handling logs, is an instrument which enables a man to greatly increase his natural leverage; but even when using a peavey, a man has to have some weight and strength in order to move logs which weigh anywhere from 500 to 2000 lbs. When it comes to picking up one end of a log which weighs several hundred pounds and helping another man to carry it a great distance, or when it comes to up-ending a lighter log, letting it fall across your shoulder, and carrying it away, then you have to have bodily strength in great quantities.

It is well known that cold air is a peptic stimulant; that is, it creates an appetite. Heavy work also creates an appetite. The combination of the two produces a kind of appetite which can be satisfied only by a large quantity of highly nourishing foods. A great deal of lumbering is done in the cold weather at high altitudes.

I claim that if you, being sickly and undersized went to a mountain lumber camp and did the kind of work I have just described, you would, in all probability, make bigger gains in a winter's work, than you could in as many years spent at calisthenics or "bending exercises." But if you went to the lumber camp in some clerical capacity, or as cook, you might gain a little in size and strength; but not much more than you would gain if you had stayed home and held the same kind of a job.

If a man ships as a "hand" on a sailing-vessel, it means that he has a job which takes the hardest kind of physical work; and if he spent his time climbing up and down the rigging, hauling on ropes in order to hoist heavy sails, and assisting in loading and unloading heavy cargoes, he would get a fine physique. If he shipped on a steamer as a wireless operator or something of that kind, he would not be likely to grow very much bigger and stronger than he was at the start. You can't transform yourself physically simply by going to a lumber camp or by going to sea. The thing that produces results is what you do after you get there. Your body will shape itself, and your muscles will develop, according to the kind of work you do; and if you know how to get that work either in the form of labor or play, you can develop yourself just as rapidly in your own home, as you can in the furthest lumber camp or most distant sea. One time, when I was tired of hearing enthusiasts talk about sleeping porches and ventilated gymnasiums and proper food and clothing, I said that if a young man would do what I told him to, he could take his exercises in a damp, unventilated cellar, that he could eat anything he pleased, smoke a pack of cigarettes a day, and drink wine or beer; and that if he got sufficient sleep and did the right kind of exercise, I could make him into a "Strong Man" in a very short space of time. Of course a man will naturally make better progress if he works under pleasant conditions; but it seems to me that sometimes there is a great deal too much attention paid to getting those pleasant conditions, and too little attention paid to the way a man works. Though you may think go, I am still talking about the same subject; which is, that great results come from great endeavor, and that great muscular development and super-strength can be acquired only by a certain kind of work. If you are willing to do that kind of work, and do it intelligently, you can get results in your own bedroom just as well as anywhere else.

In the stories mentioned in the first part of this chapter, it is noticed the hero's friends always exclaimed about the difference in the size of his chest and shoulders. They did not say, "My, your legs have gotten big!" or, "What wonderful arms you have!"; but, "What a chest you have!" and, "My, you have spread out around the shoulders!" In chapter 8, I described one exercise which will increase the size of the chest by increasing the size of the rib-box; and I urged you to practice that exercise even if you are not interested in the subject of great strength. I am convinced that the kind of chest which gives plenty of lung room, is the one which a super-strong man must have. I know that the average man can greatly increase his vitality and make himself somewhat bigger and stronger, merely by increasing the size of the chest, even if he does not take special exercises for the other parts of the body. Therefore, I believe that if a man actually wishes to "make himself over," the first and most important thing is to increase the size of the rib-box.

In the fall of 1923, I wrote an article in the Strength magazine in which I made a comparison of British and American lifters. I pointed out the fact that while England had a large number of first-class lifters among the smaller men, they had very few first-class big men. Also, that in this country, we had a great number of "Strong Men" in the heavy-weight division, whereas, England had only one or two. This article excited a good deal of discussion in the English sporting papers; and in their comments, they tried to make it seem as though I favored bulk and brute strength, in preference to lifting skill. That is not quite the truth. I cheerfully admit that I do find it a much more interesting and, I believe, a more valuable work to develop men, than to develop lifters.

One English writer admitted the shortage of first-class heavyweights in Great Britain; but claimed that they "did not breed big men in England." Now I have seen plenty of big Englishmen; tall, broad-shouldered, deep-chested fellows, who could easily be trained into high-grade amateur "Strong Men." Some of the most famous "Strong Men" in history are

Scotchmen. From Ireland, there come a large number of gigantic weight-throwers, and I cannot believe that large men are scarce in England. But perhaps none of their big chaps become interested in bar-bell work. My point is that the breeding has but little to do with the cultivation of super-strength, and that individual training and individual effort can overcome the handicaps of heredity. A man whose parents were short in stature, is not likely to become very tall, himself; but one does not have to be a very tall man in order to be a big man. A perfectly developed man of 5 feet 8 inches, will weigh anywhere from 165 to 185 lbs., according to the size of his bones. Steinborn stands less than 5 feet 8 inches, and weighs 215 lbs. in a hard condition. Adolph Nordquest, who weighs about as much, stands 5 feet 9 inches. Certainly there must be thousands of men of that height in England.

In the article referred to, I mentioned some cases of phenomenal growth which have come under my observation. One English authority claimed that no mart could make the increases I cited "unless he had the bodily framework on which to build"; apparently overlooking the fact that even at the age of thirty, it is possible to make a marked change in the bony framework of the body. I do not mean that you can make the bones longer or increase your height, or the length of your arms and legs; but I positively have seen cases where the bones became thicker and stronger, although such cases are somewhat rare.

If you examine a man's skeleton, the length of the bones will give you an accurate idea of how long that man's arms and legs were. The hipbones, which constitute what we call the "pelvic basin," will show you how wide his hips were. The size of the rib-box and the articulation of the shoulders, give an idea, (although not an accurate one,) of his shoulder-breadth. I do not claim that it is possible, after maturity, to make a man's hips wider by promoting the growth of the bones of the pelvis; although by properly developing the muscles of the upper thigh and hip region, it is possible to make them an inch or two wider.

While it is not possible to make the ribs, themselves, any longer, it is distinctly possible to increase the size of the rib-box by lengthening the cartilages which connect the ribs with the breast-bone. By the time most men are twenty-five years old, these cartilages have entirely lost their original elasticity; and if a man of that age has a flat chest, he gets the idea that he is condemned to have a flat chest for the rest of his life. By doing certain exercises, notably the one illustrated in Fig. 42, and combining them with special breathing, it is possible, in a few months' time, to convert a flat chest into a high-arched chest. The breast-bone, which has originally been flat, assumes a distinct outward curve. The breast-bone is made up of three sections, and its shape determines the appearance and size of your chest. The lower two sections are joined together so tightly that they seem to be one bone; but the upper section is more loosely joined to the other two. However, a high-arched chest is more dependent upon the shape of the rib-box than upon the amount of curve (or lack of curve), in the breast-bone. The round-shouldered man almost invariably has a flat chest; while a man with a flat back, almost invariably has a high-arched chest.

Mr. Arthur Thomson, the eminent anatomist says, "After the age of twenty-five, when all the bones are fully ossified and the figure set, any form of exercise will have but little influence on the form of the thorax, except that it stimulates a more healthy respiration. Yet we cannot but admit the effect which the exercise has had on the man, for he appears now with braced-up figure and square shoulders. The increase in breadth of the chest is not due to any marked increase in the capacity or form of the chest-wall, but is due almost entirely to the increase in size of the muscles, brought about by exercise. As has been shown, some of these muscles lie between the blade-bone and the chest-wall, and one can readily understand how any increase in the thickness of these layers will tend to push upwards and outwards the blade-bone from the chest-wall, and so impart to the shoulders that squareness which is so desirable in the male figure.

According to Mr. Thomson, it would seem hopeless to alter the size or shape of the rib-box after the age of twenty-five, and yet I have seen men of thirty-five increase their chest measurements six, eight, ten, and, in one case, twelve inches. Such an amount of increase cannot be made simply by developing the muscles which overlay the ribs. The circumference of a circle is, roughly, three times its diameter. If you were to develop the pectoral muscles on the chest so that they were one inch thicker than before, and developed the back muscles so that they were one inch thicker, it would mean that the whole chest would be two inches thicker, and that would account for only a six-inch difference in the girth of the chest. The pectoral muscles can be made very big and thick, and the muscles across the back of the shoulders are capable of high development; but I do not believe that any of these muscles can be made two inches thicker.

Note that Mr. Thomson speaks only of the increase in the breadth of the chest. When you increase the size of the rib-box by promoting the elasticity of the rib-cartilages, the chest becomes deeper from front to back. The difference between a very shallow chest and a very deep one, is just the difference between weakness and super-strength. In converting a small and shallow rib-box into a big, deep and roomy one, part of the increase is obtained by developing certain muscles on the outside of the chest, which have a tendency to lift the ribs; and another part comes from the pressure from within, furnished by the growing lungs.

A man possessed of super-strength almost invariably has lungs of great size and high quality, and the upper part of his lungs is of larger size than in the ordinary individual. This is because most of them are adepts at costal breathing. (When it comes to breathing methods, I am an ardent disciple of the late Edwin Checkley.) In the chapter devoted to developing the upper-back muscles, I mentioned only one or two of the larger muscles. Besides these, there are a number of smaller muscles, some of which help to control the movement of the arm, and others, the movement of the shoulder-blade and the ribs. By developing those muscles you will help to make the shoulders square and to increase the width of the back. A man can have a big chest measurement without having any particular development of the pectoral muscles on the breast. Even if those muscles are of moderate size, the big-chested man is sure to be very wide across the upper-back, from one armpit to the other, and it is around that part of the body the tape is passed when taking the chest measurement. If, in addition to a wide upper-back, a man has a deep rib-box, the chest measurement becomes phenomenal. (When I say a "deep chest" or a "deep rib-box," I mean deep from front to back; that is, from the breastbone to the spine.)

When my English critic said "it was impossible to make enormous gains unless one had the bodily framework on which to build," he ignored this possibility of increasing the size of the chest itself. In my article I mentioned the case of a boy who had increased his chest measurement 7 inches in one month by the use of bar-bells. It would have been utterly impossible to gain that much just by developing the muscles on the upper body, because that would have meant making the chest muscles and the back muscles an inch thicker than before. So much development can't possibly be gained in thirty days' time; but since the boy referred to did actually make the 7-inch increase, at least half of that gain was due to an increase in the size of the rib-box. When the lad started his normal chest measurement was 29 inches. By developing the muscles on the outside of the chest he could possibly have brought his chest measurement up to 38 or 39 inches by a couple of years' steady work. All this gain would have been muscular, and his original framework would have remained the same. At the end of thirty days he had a considerably bigger bodily framework than at the start of his training, and with that framework, by developing the exterior muscles, he might have eventually gotten up to a 40-inch chest measurement; but as it happened, he continued at the exercises which expanded the chest, kept on increasing the size of his frame, and at the end of the year had a 43-inch chest, making a total gain of 14 inches in the year.

You may object that this boy was only seventeen years old when he started, and that therefore he was still growing. That is unquestionably true. If he had never exercised at all, it is quite likely that his chest would have increased from 29 to 32 inches in one year by natural growth; but at that, his chest never would have been more than 36 or 37 inches at the age of twenty-one, because he was originally built on slender lines. I do not merely claim that he enlarged and improved his bodily framework. I know it.

If I had the space I could tell you of almost as remarkable gains made by men who had passed the age where growth is supposed to stop. I saw a man of thirty years increase his chest measurement from 35 to 44 inches in one year; and during that time his shoulders became nearly 4 inches broader. I know a man, Professor Lange, who, at the age of thirty, started to practice the exercises which I have described in chapters 8 and 10. He had been interested in athletics all his life, and at the age of eighteen his chest measured only 30 inches. At the age of thirty his twelve years' practice had increased his chest to 36 inches. By specializing on chest development he increased the measurement within the next few years to 48 inches. When his chest grew, he grew all over. So far as I know, he did not grow any taller; but the development of his back, his shoulders, his arms and his legs kept pace with the growth of his chest. After he was thirty his upper arms increased from 13½ inches to 18½ inches, and his thighs from 21 inches to 28 inches. Even his forearms and the calves of his legs increased at the same rate, and the development of those parts of the body is supposed to be limited by the size of the bones below the elbow and knee. If that man had had a really big frame, it is impossible that his chest would have measured as little as 36 inches at the age of thirty. The fact that he has almost the deepest chest on record is positive proof that he made the rib-box larger. Therefore, he deliberately and successfully altered his own bodily framework. I regret that I cannot show you his pictures. He will not allow them to be published, although some pictures of him did appear in the Strength magazine in 1919 and 1920.

I could go on multiplying the number of these cases. The three I have just mentioned are exceptional; but they prove what can be done. For a bar-bell user to gain from 4 to 6 inches in chest measurement during the first three months is so common a happening that it is hardly worth while mentioning.

There is an immense difference between the shape of a man who has thus developed himself and the shape of a man who has increased his size just by thickening and developing the muscles. There is a certain relation between the size of the arms and chest in a well- proportioned man; in fact, there should be a fixed relation between the sizes of all parts of the body. A bar-bell user who has a 17- inch upper arm usually has a 44- or 45-inch chest and a 24-inch thigh. If his upper arm is 16 inches, his chest is 43 to 44 inches, and his thigh about 23½ inches. I have seen professional gymnasts, especially Roman-ring performers, with 16½ inch upper arms and only 39-inch chest and 20-inch thighs.

That alone explains why the average bar-bell user so greatly excels the average gymnast in the matter of bodily strength.

As I said in a previous chapter, an increase in the size of the rib-box is always accompanied by a corresponding and proportionate increase in the breadth of the shoulders; which is puzzling, because the collar bones do not seem to become any longer, although the shoulder blades becomes wider spaced; that is, set further apart. A man with a 36-inch chest will have shoulders about 17 inches in width. A 40-inch chest usually means shoulders about 19 inches wide; whereas, a "Strong Man," that is, an individual with super- strength, may have a 46-inch chest, with shoulders that are fully 23 inches across.

The deltoid muscles lie on the points of the shoulders, but no man could increase the width of the shoulders from 17 to 23 inches by making each deltoid three inches thicker; and one would have to do that in order to add six inches to the shoulder-breadth. While Mr. Lange's chest was increasing from 36 to 48 inches, his shoulders became six inches wider, notwithstanding the fact that a large part of the gain in chest girth was due to the deepening of the chest box. When a novelist describes his "Strong Man" character, he is apt to say, "His broad shoulders and deep chest gave indication of his enormous physical strength." It seems to be an accepted idea that depth of chest is a sign of great natural vitality, and that broad shoulders indicate the possession of great natural power. (That is a case where the popular or general view is the correct one.) I go further and say that you can deliberately make your chest deeper and your shoulders broader, and that as you do so your natural vitality and strength will increase to an extent that will go a long way towards putting you in the class of the super-strong.

The bigger rib-box will mean more lung room, and big, high-quality lungs make not only for endurance, but for vitality and driving power. The deep-chested (and therefore big-lunged) man will sustain without fatigue a series of exertions, any one of which would exhaust a shallow-chested, small-lunged man.

The gain in the width of the shoulders is accompanied by a gain in sheer arm and shoulder power, which is due to the greater and more advantageous leverages. If you can make your shoulders broader by making your rib-box bigger, you will find that you are possessed of an entirely new kind of strength, even if you pay little attention to developing the muscles on the points of the shoulders and the front and back of the upper-body. If, in addition, you can properly develop those muscles, you will become so strong that you will be a source of pride to your friends and a terror to your enemies.

It is a great advantage to a "Strong Man" to have fairly wide hips; but the size of the hip-bones which constitute the "pelvic-basin," cannot be materially altered after full maturity, as the individual bones are firmly welded together. Nevertheless, the shape and power of the hips can be greatly improved and increased by the exercises in Chapters 2 and 4 for the thighs and lower back.

The "fashionable" figure is that of a man with wide shoulders and narrow hips. Novelists, and some writers on art subjects, seem to think that small hips add elegance to the figure; whereas, narrow hips are a sign of immaturity. At present, women have such a craze for narrow hips, that the corset, which in other days constricted the waist, has been extended downward so as to act as a compressor of the soft flesh around the hips. Reason? They think that small hips make them look more youthful. "The boyish figure!" That is their present ideal. In men, unusually narrow hips are often a sign of arrested development. The hips and shoulders should grow wider between the ages of 18 and 23, after the full height has been attained. All of you are familiar with the spectacle of a youth "broadening out" as he approaches maturity.

I have always found it much easier to give perfect proportions to a beginner with good hips and comparatively narrow shoulders than to the beginner who has fair shoulders and poor hips. Qualify that, by saying my idea of perfect proportions, for I believe that a man is best built for bodily strength, when the girth of the hips is three or four inches less than the girth of the normal chest, {not the expanded chest). Saxon, Steinborn and Hackenschmidt have wide hips. Sandow, Walter Donald and men of their type have hips that are smaller in proportion to their chests. Undoubtedly, the Sandow-Donald type is more pleasing to the eye; but the Saxon-Steinborn type have more sheer bodily power.

Let us see how it works out. In the Strength Magazine, we held a discussion as to the proper relative size of the hips and thighs. It appeared that in most men who combine great strength and great development, the thigh girth was about 60 percent of the girth of the hips. (Both measurements taken at the largest part). For example; Sandow's hips measured 39 inches, and his thigh 23.7 inches. The thigh measurement is almost exactly 60 percent of the girth of the hips. Now Sandow's thigh-development was a thing to wonder at, and when you look at his picture, it seems impossible that a man could have more powerfully developed thighs with such trim hips; yet I have seen men with smaller hips and bigger thighs; for instance, Mr. Fred Rohde, Fig. 83, has a 25-inch thigh and hips measuring only 35½ inches around. I could name several others whose thigh measurement is more than 60 percent as large as the hip measurement.

The foregoing reads almost as though I were trying to dodge the issue and to claim that great development could be acquired without changing the size of the bony framework of the hips. The hips may not actually get any wider; but unquestionably, they seem to get bigger as the chest grows in size. Look at the picture of Mr. Frank Dilks on Fig 84. This man was extremely slender before he started to train, and the fact that he was above the average height, accentuated his slenderness. Since he had only a 36-inch chest and a 10-inch upper-arm, his hips couldn't have been much more than 35 inches around. This picture of him was taken after one year of bar-bell exercises, and during that time, his chest had increased to 44 inches, and his thigh, from 20 inches to 24 inches. What his hips measure at present, I do not know; but surely they must be at least 40 inches around. While in the photograph they appear noticeably smaller than his chest, they are not so small as to give any impression of weakness. This is because Mr. Dilks, by practicing heavy exercises for the legs, developed the muscles on the upper part of the thighs where they emerge into the hips.

When Mr. Lange started at thirty years, with his 36-inch chest, his hips were of a size that corresponded to his chest. While his chest was increasing from 36 to 48 inches, his hip measurement increased about 7 inches, and his pictures in my private collection, show that at present the difference in size between his chest and hips is just about the same proportion as the difference between Sandow's chest and hips.

The important thing is that as your rib-box increases in size, the hips either grow, or seem to grow, in proportion; for I have never seen a man with a really big rib-box, who had inadequate hips. Perhaps the explanation is that the big-chested man can add to his muscular development with comparative ease; but that does seem to entirely cover the case, because there is very little muscle on the sides of the hips. It is possible to increase the hip measurement by developing the muscles which compose the buttocks, but that does not mean that you make your hips any wider.

In Chapters 2 and 4, I recommend that the beginner at bar-bell work start with exercises for the thighs and the lower part of the back. The strength of the lower-back is intimately connected and controlled by the size of the hips and the development and strength of the upper-legs. Some writers seem to think it indelicate to refer to the hips, especially to those muscles which compose the buttocks, and which are such an important link in the chain of muscles which hold the body erect. Big arms are spectacular; a big chest is almost indispensable; powerful legs are a great help; but to the man seeking super-strength, one great requisite is strong loins.

No matter how big your upper-arm is, you cannot exert the full strength of that arm unless the muscles of your shoulder are even more powerful than the arm-muscles. No matter how big your thighs are, they cannot exert their full strength unless the hips and loins are even stronger. That is why I was so particular in Chapter 4, to give you exercises which develop the hips and loins in connection with the leg muscles.

The most striking example I have ever seen of strong loins and hips, is Henry Steinborn. This man trained himself to a point where he could take 400 lbs. on his shoulders and do the squat many times in succession, as in Fig. 27.

His constant practice of the quick lifts had given him immense power in the loins. In lifting heavy bar-bells from the floor to the shoulder, he could show more energy than any athlete on record. He could lift more weight clean from floor to the shoulders than any other athlete in the world; and in that style of lifting, the power that raises the weight from the floor comes from the thighs and the loins. In writing an article about this man, I said one stamp of his foot, he could crush the life out of any creature smaller than a tiger. His strength of leg and loin was the explanation of this unparalleled quickness of movement. In jumping, springing and quick lifting, the impulse comes from the hips; and Steinborn, who weighed 215 lbs., could move his body about with more rapidity and greater ease than even such famous fancy dancers as Nijinsky and Mordkin.

In a later chapter, I will say a few words about the connection between loin strength and general vitality.

CHAPTER XVII

HANDS, WRISTS AND FOREARMS

Golfers, baseball players, poloists and tennis players, all recognize the great value of strong wrists. Weak wrists are a handicap even in such light forms of athletics as I have named. A "Strong Man" with weak wrists would be unthinkable. One thing about handling bar-bells is that you get strong wrists, whether you want them or not. In almost every exercise that is performed with weights, you have to hold the bar-bell in your hands. Even when performing an exercise for the back and legs, like the one shown in Fig. 10, you develop a great gripping power in the hands. In fact, when doing this exercise with 75 lbs. the beginner's fingers will commence to slip before the back muscles themselves feel the effect of the weight.

Nevertheless, most aspirants for super-strength spend some of their time in still further increasing the strength of the hands and forearms. There are no muscles in the wrist itself; only bones and tendons. Therefore, the only way to make your wrist stronger is to increase the size and strength of the muscles in the hands and forearms. As your wrist gets stronger, your hands will become thicker and more compact, even if they do not get wider and longer. If you work for super-strength, you simply cannot keep a lady-like pair of hands.

(George Washington was supposed to have the strongest arm of any man in the Continental Army. After his death a cast was made from his right hand, which shows that his hand was very much bigger than the average. Washington was a big man and apparently the best athlete of his time. He made a record of 23 feet in a running broad-jump, and this record stood until Malcolm Ford beat it by 4 inches, around 1880. Judging by the size of his hand, Washington must have had a forearm which measured over 13 inches.)

In order to fully develop the power of the wrist it is necessary to practice (a) gripping exercises for the hands, (b) twisting exercises for the wrists, and (c) forearm exercises for that part of the forearm near the elbow. The popular idea is that the way to get forearm development is to clinch the fist tightly and then to bend the wrist; but this gives only a partial development of the forearm. There is nothing which develops the gripping power of the hands so much as does using bar-bells with thick handlebars. When you use a thin handlebar, the fingers encircle the handle, and so there is not much strain on the grip. It is necessary to use thin handles in many kinds of actual lifting, and therefore some lifters make a practice of using a thick handled bar-bell or dumbbell in some of their exercises. If the handle is more than 2 inches in diameter the fingers will not lap around it, and consequently the lifter develops an incredible pinching power in his thumbs and fingers.

One very good exercise for strengthening the wrist is to take a pair of light dumbbells, hold them by the hands, stretch your arms out to the sides, and then describe circles with the free ends of the bells. You should use dumbbells which have the mushroom- shaped end, and you should hold them as in Fig. 85. A pair of 5-pounders is enough to start with, and after a short time you will be able to do the exercise with a pair of 10-pounders; and when you have gotten so that you can use a pair of 15-pounders, you will notice a great increase in your gripping power and in your wrist strength.

But even that will not bring the forearm to the highest state of development. Some of the muscles in the forearm are attached at the lower end to the bones of the wrist, and at the upper end to the bones of the forearm. Therefore, every time you bend your arms against resistance, you develop those forearm muscles. Most of you consider that chinning the bar is simply a biceps exercise; but it develops the forearms almost as much as the upper arms. When you curl a heavy dumbbell with one hand, the forearm muscles get more work than in chinning. Examine Fig. 73 and you can plainly see one of the forearm muscles which helps bend the arm. (It makes the line which runs from the base of the thumb to the bottom of the biceps.)

The very best forearm exercise is the one invented by George Zottman. He used to do it with a pair of 50-lb. dumbbells, and you can start it with a pair of 20-pounders. Stand erect, with the arms hanging at the sides. Then bend your right arm and bring the bell up in front of your chest, with the palm of the hand up and the wrist bent strongly inward. Bring the hand still further up until it is in front of the right shoulder, and then rotate your forearm until the palm is front, and then lower the bell slowly (with knuckles up) until the arm is again hanging at the side. The right hand describes a complete circle. When your right hand is in front of your shoulder, start your left hand coming up. Both hands work at the same time, but as the right hand is coming down the left hand is coming up, and vice versa. Fig. 86 shows the left hand (knuckles up) on the way down, and the right hand (palm up) on the way up. This exercise develops all the muscles in the forearm. By gripping the dumbbells firmly, you develop the muscles of the hand; the muscles which bend the wrist inward are developed as you raise the bells; and the muscles on the outside of the forearm (which bend the wrist outward) are developed as you lower the bells. The elbows should be kept close to the sides throughout the whole exercise.

Zottman's forearm strength is phenomenal. At one of our exhibitions he was acting as judge. One lift had been completed, and a couple of assistants were dismantling a very heavy bar-bell of the plate-loading type. (The kind shown in Fig. 14.) The biggest plates on this bell weighed 50 lbs. each and were 11 inches in diameter and 2 inches thick. In order to carry one of these plates, the average man would hold it in both hands. One of the assistants was justly proud of the strength of his grip. He stood two of these plates on edge, gripped one in each hand by the upper edges, walked over and placed them at Zottman's feet and said, "George, can you do that?" Zottman immediately leaned over, gripped the plates by the top edges, just as the other man had done, and then stood up straight and "muscled out" the plates, one to each side. Then he grinned at the other man and said, "And can you do that?" (Zottman was 50 years old at that time, and the only two men I know of who could have duplicated this stunt were Joe Nordquest and the English lifter, Vansart.) Any bar-bell exercise which develops the biceps muscle also develops the forearm. The ordinary two-arm curl, shown in Fig. 72, is a great forearm developer, if you are careful to bend the wrists inward as you raise the bell. To develop the outside of the forearms by curling, you have to hold the bell by the over-grip, knuckles up, as shown in Fig. 87. You can curl nearly twice as much with the under-grip as with the over-grip, just the same as you can chin yourself twice as often on a horizontal bar when you hold the palms of your hands towards you as when you hold the palms of your hands away from you.

One of the greatest tests of forearm strength is to curl a thick bar with the over-grip. Once I bought a round steel bar, about feet long and 2 inches thick, which weighed 65 lbs. To do a two-arm curl with this steel bar was a cinch if you used the under-grip; but when you tried to curl it with the over-grip, the bar would slip out of your hands when the arms were bent half way. Lots of lifters who could do a back-hand curl easily with a thin-handled 100-lb. bar-bell, utterly failed to do the same thing with the thick 65-lb. bar. Anton Matysek could do it easily; Juvenal, the oarsman, could do it with even greater ease; and Zottman simply played with it. In order to curl the bar successfully, it was necessary to have tremendous gripping power in the hands and great strength in the muscles on the outside of the forearm; but the gripping power was more important. This stunt interested me so much that I had a special bar made, which consisted of a 4-inch pipe, and from each end of that pipe projected a 1-inch iron rod. We could load up the handle by slipping plates over the 1-inch rods. At one of our exhibitions Matysek demonstrated the exercise while I explained the principles involved. Joe Nordquest, who was present, demanded that he be allowed to try his strength, and soon there was a competition in progress. According to our rules, the lifter had to stand bolt upright and keep his elbows at his sides, in order to prevent him from getting any advantage from a swing of the body or a movement of the upper arms. One of the two claimed that the other one was not playing fair; so before each attempt we bound a belt around their upper arms, as in Fig. 88. Matysek finally won with 88 lbs., which was harder than curling a 1½-inch-handled 125-lb. bar-bell. Tests like that interest me far more than lifts in which a man's ability is dependent on skill as well as strength.

It is very important to develop your forearm to the limit, because the bigger your forearm gets, the bigger your upper arm can get. In fact, if you properly develop your forearms and the deltoid muscles on the point of the shoulder, your upper arms will develop themselves. If you have time only for a little forearm exercise, use the Zottman exercise, or two-hand curling in preference to the exercise shown in Fig. 85.

You remember that when I talked to you about the back and legs, I compared them to the two leaves of a hinge and said that both leaves must be of equal strength, and that the strength of the small of the back was influenced by the strength of the muscles on the back of the thighs, and vice versa. Exactly this same principal applies to the forearm and the biceps. The power with which you can bend your arm depends not on the biceps alone, but on the biceps plus the forearm. If you can grasp this principle, you will at once understand why it is that while devotees of light exercise rarely succeed in getting forearm larger than 11½-inches around, a bar-bell user is not satisfied with a forearm which measures much less than 13 inches.

Extreme finger strength can be developed by lifting weights from the ground with one finger at a time as in Fig. 89. That is a rather dangerous exercise, because if you make an attempt at a weight which is too heavy, it is possible to snap a tendon. It is perfectly possible to develop the finger strength to the greatest possible extent by using the whole hand, rather than one finger at a time. One-finger lifting is a favorite stunt with exhibitionists; but those men commonly use a prepared grip of such a shape that once the finger is inserted in the grip, it is almost impossible for any amount of weight to straighten out the finger. Such lifts are interesting from an exhibition stand-point; but they have little or nothing to do with the creation of strength, which is the subject in which we are concerned.

PLATE 55

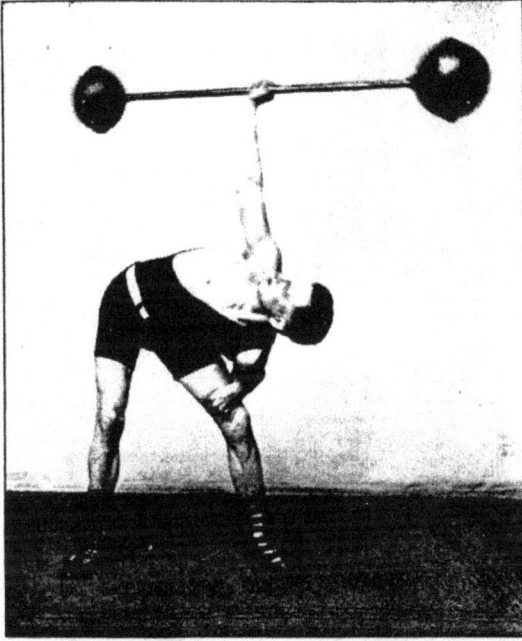

Fig. 115

Plate 55, Figure 115 (above). The lifting arm has finally been straightened by pushing hard against the weight with the hand. In order to stand erect, the lifter will bend the right leg at the knee, and squat under the weight, as that makes it easier to come to the upright position

Fig. 116

Figure 116 (below). An effort to press 220 lbs., which was unsuccessful, because the lifter failed to use his left arm as a support

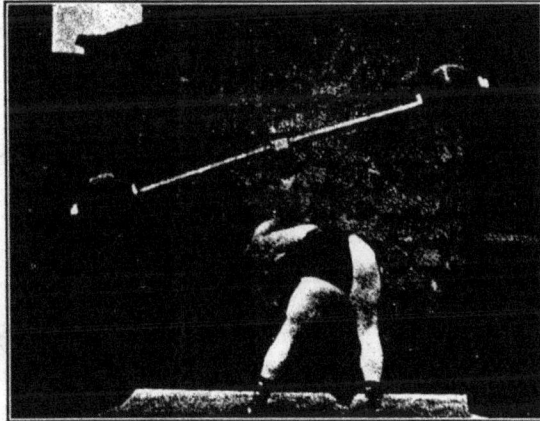

173

PLATE 56

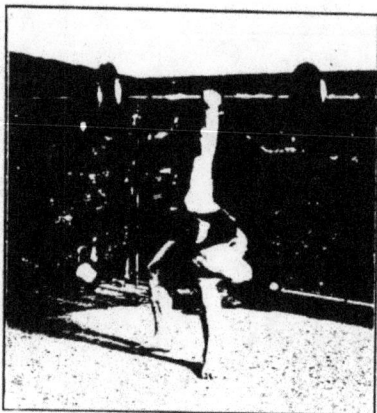

Fig. 117

Plate 56. Figure 117 (above).
Owen Carr making a "Bent
Press" in perfect style with
230 lbs.

Fig. 118

Figure 118 (below). Roy L.
Smith making a press with
173 lbs. His record is 245
lbs.

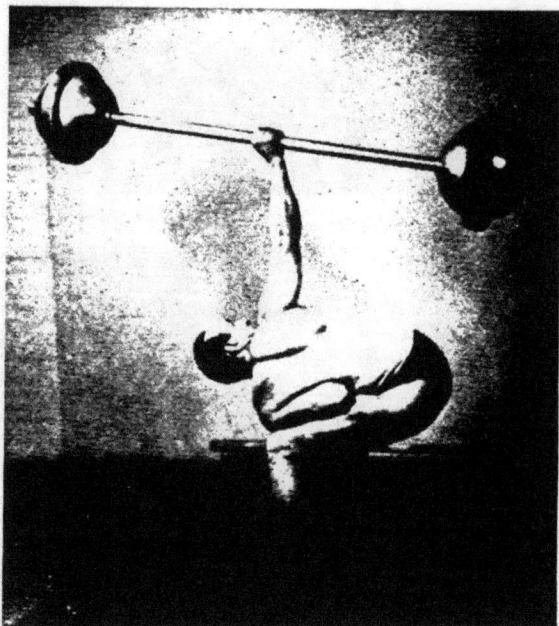

174

PLATE 57

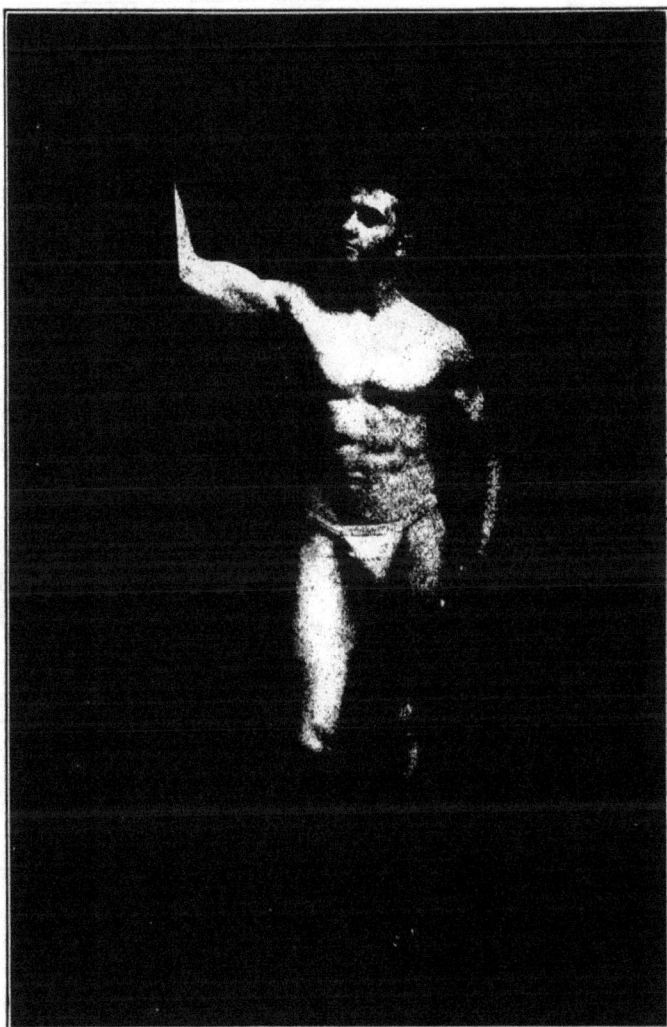

Fig. 119

Plate 57, Figure 119. Matysek standing at ease, with all his muscles
relaxed, proving that a lifter's muscles are as smooth as those of
any other athlete.

PLATE 58

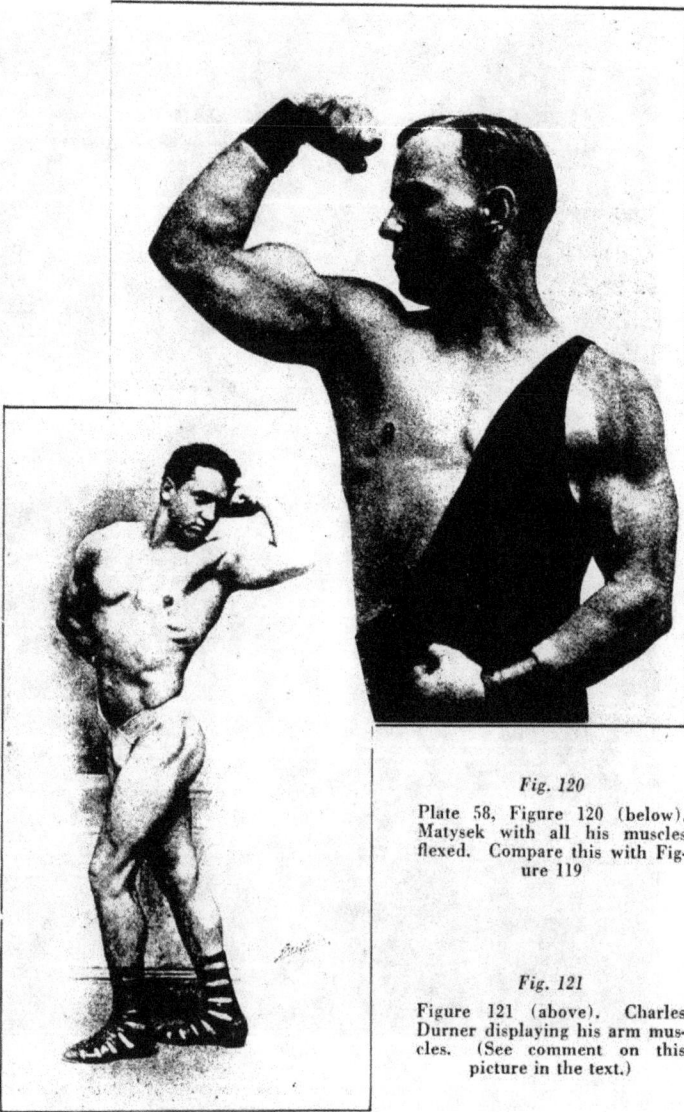

Fig. 120

Plate 58, Figure 120 (below).
Matysek with all his muscles
flexed. Compare this with Figure 119

Fig. 121

Figure 121 (above). Charles
Durner displaying his arm muscles. (See comment on this
picture in the text.)

PLATE 59

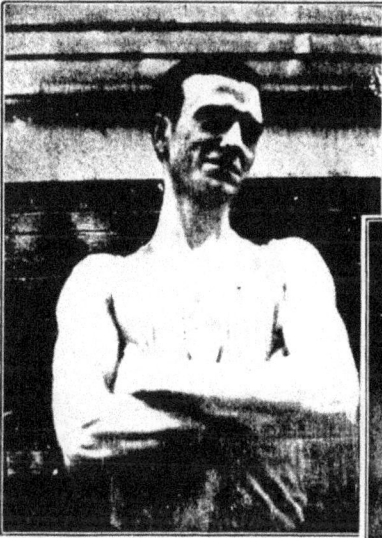

Fig. 122

Plate 59, Figure 122 (above).
J. Woodrow before he started
training.

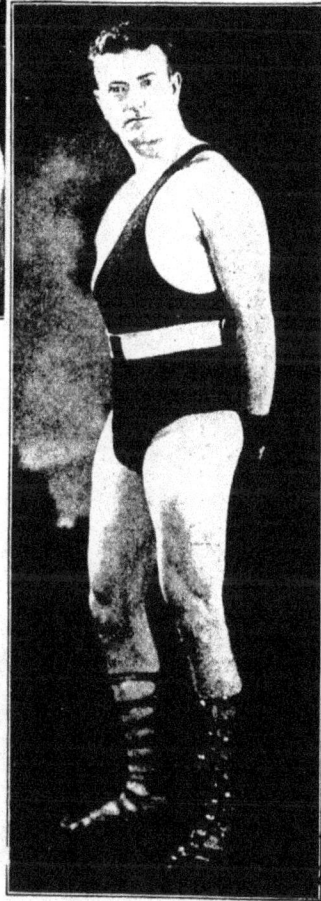

Fig. 123

Figure 123 (below). Woodrow
after having practiced for eighteen
months with an adjustable bar-bell.
This man's improvement was not
merely in the size and shape of his
muscles. His chest increased in
size, his shoulders grew broader,
and his gain in health and condition is demonstrated by the improved appearance of the face and
neck

PLATE 60

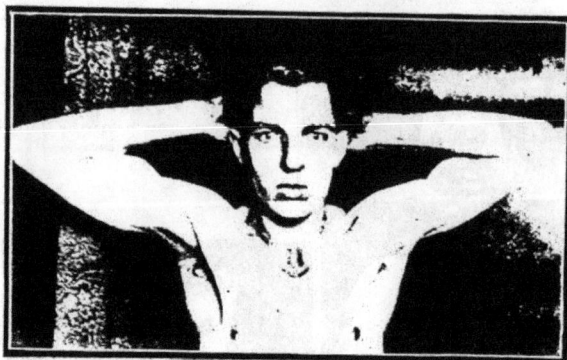

Fig. 124

Plate 60, Figure 124 (above), A. P. Hedlund, at the time he started to train with bar-bells.

Fig. 125

Figure 125 (below). Hedlund after eighteen months' training. During this time his chest increased 8 inches and his arm 3 inches in girth.

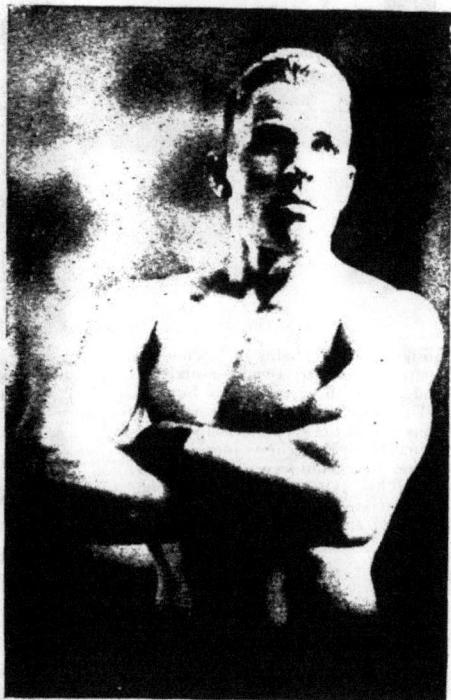

178

PLATE 61

Fig. 126

Plate 61, Figure
126 (above).
Robert Ruckstool
after six months'
training with a
bar-bell

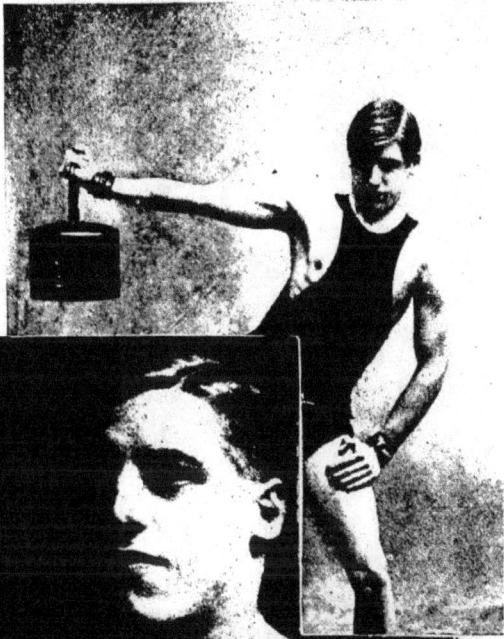

Fig. 127

Figure 127 (be-
low). Ruckstool
one year later

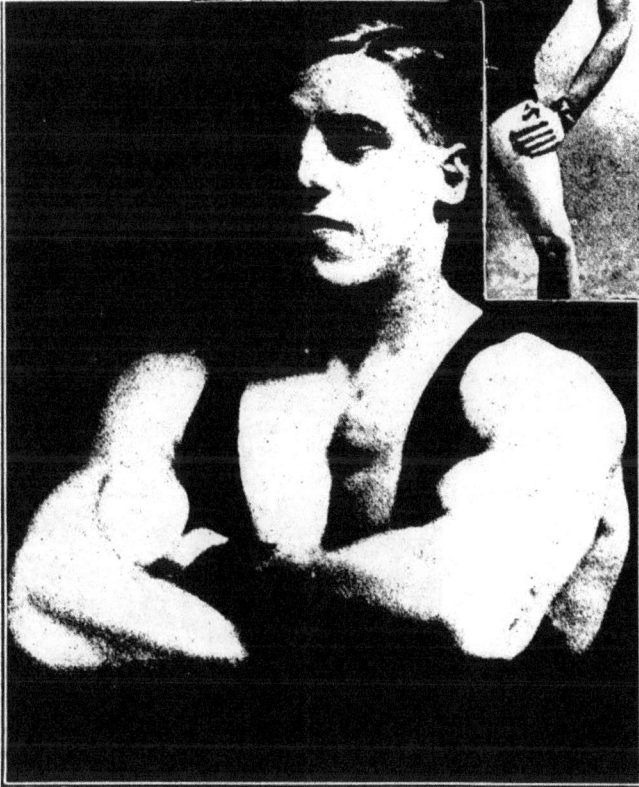

PLATE 62

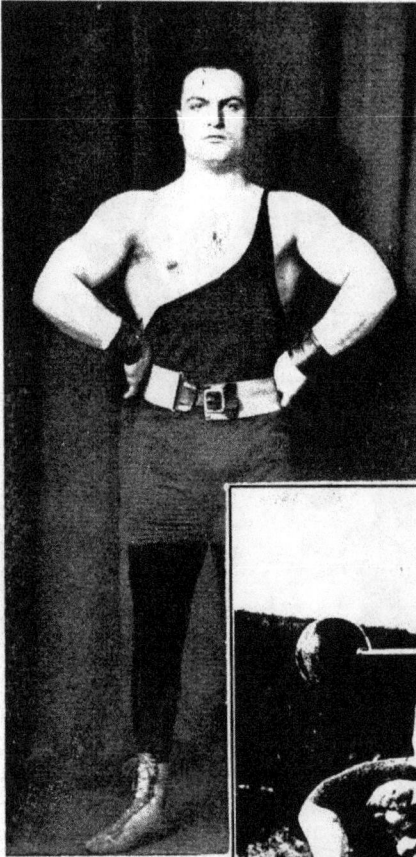

Fig. 128

Plate 62, Figure 128 (above), Robert Snyder, a great lifter, who weighs 145 lbs., is a small-boned man with a wonderful muscular development. Although his wrist measures only 6½ inches, the girth of his upper arm is 14¾ inches.

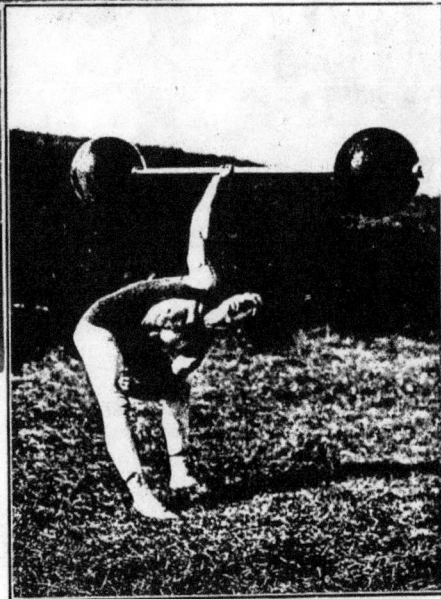

Fig. 129

Figure 129 (below), Snyder making a "Bent Press." His record in this style is 225 lbs.

CHAPTER XVIII

WHERE DOES IT ALL COME FROM?

Bar-bell lifting is a fascinating sport. Almost everyone who tries it becomes intensely interested. It seems to be a case of "once a lifter, always a lifter!" I know men who began using bar-bells twenty years ago, and who are just as much interested today in feats of strength, and in subjects related to muscular development, as they were on the day they started. But the matter of body-building, health-improvement and muscular-development, is much more important than lifting records.

When a man first starts to practice with adjustable bar-bells, it takes two or three weeks to break himself in to the new kind of work; that is, to learn the positions and to accustom his muscles to the more vigorous contractions. As soon as he commences to increase the weight used in the exercises, his body grows in size and weight in almost direct proportion to the increased weight used. His chest gets bigger, his shoulders broader, and his arms and legs commence to put on muscle.

Now where does it all come from? If a man at the start has a 12-inch upper arm, and that arm increases to 14 inches in girth at the end of three months and 16 inches in girth at the end of six months, it means that he has almost doubled the amount of muscular tissue in the upper arm. The upper-arm bone would not have grown any longer, so all the increase of the arm is in girth and muscular contents. When you say that your arm has increased from 12 to 16 inches in girth, it sounds as though it increased only one-third in size; but if you remember that an arm of 12-inch girth means a cross section of about 11½ square inches, and that an arm of 16-inch girth means a cross section of more than 21 square inches, you will see that your arm has nearly doubled in bulk. Since the upper-arm bone is no thicker than before, all that increased bulk is solid muscular tissue; and that means that each individual muscle in the upper arm is nearly twice as big as before.

A muscle is made up of a bundle of fibrous tissue. So the question is, "Do the fibers in your muscles become thicker; do they become more numerous; or both?"

When you exercise a muscle, part of the tissue is broken down; and when you rest after exercise, the broken-down tissue is replaced and reconstructed by fresh material supplied by the blood. That means that in order to grow, the muscle must be well-nourished as well as thoroughly exercised. The greatest value of bar-bell exercise is its undoubted effect in promoting the vigor of your digestive and assimilative processes; and that brings me around to the question of dieting.

I am personally acquainted with dozens of professional "Strong Men," and hundreds of amateur lifters. Furthermore, I have examined the measurement charts and reports of thousands of bar-bell users whom I have never met personally. Among all those thousands, I can't recall a dozen individuals who are "diet faddists." If you use bar-bells regularly—that is, two or three hours a week—you will get such an appetite that you can digest, assimilate and build yourself up on just the same bill-of- fare that the rest of your family eat. It is positively not necessary to confine your diet to certain articles of food; such as cereal, fruit, nuts or vegetables.

If you are a thin man and wish to grow bigger and heavier, as well as stronger, you must satisfy the appetite which you have created by exercise. You have to eat enough to repair the ordinary wear and tear of the day, and on top of that, you have to eat enough more to grow on. During the time that your chest is increasing 6 inches, your arms 2 inches, and your thighs 3 inches in girth, you will eat like a growing schoolboy. Why not?

182

The boy is growing rapidly, and so will you be growing rapidly. You cannot add to your size and bodily weight if you deliberately restrict your diet, either in quantity or to particular foods.

The human teeth prove that a man can eat either meat, vegetables or grain, and it seems to me that the ordinary individual will grow faster on just the mixed diet that the average housewife provides.

Occasionally, a bar-bell user will write to me and say that he is not growing as fast as he expected to, and he will finish up his letter by saying, "And I can't understand this, because I am careful to eat properly." An investigation usually develops the fact that his idea of eating "properly," is to have the juice of an orange and some cereal for breakfast; some vegetables, toast, fruit and nuts for the noon meal; and that his evening meal is a sort of a combination of the other two. I can readily see that such a diet might be very helpful in the case of a stout, middle-aged individual who had grown very fat through lack of exercise, whose digestive processes were debilitated, and who wished to reduce his weight by many pounds. But no one could build up real size and muscular development on such a diet.

It seems so easy when some one tells you that you can make yourself bigger and stronger just by eating some foods and avoiding other foods. Of course the thing is possible. By eating a malt preparation, either in a liquid or solid form, a scrawny individual can add 20 to 30 lbs. to his weight in a comparatively short time; but then a beer-drinker can do exactly the same thing. In both cases it means that you make a gain of, say, 20 lbs., most of which is soft flesh which you have to carry around, instead of an extra 20 lbs. of muscle which would help carry you around. It is easy for you to come back and say, "But that can't be entirely true. I know a man who is very strong who eats nothing except vegetables," or it may be "nothing except fruit and nuts." My answer to that is that if that man ate plenty of a mixed diet, including meat at least once a day, he would be even stronger than he is now on his limited diet. The amount of strength you will eventually possess will be more dependent on the kind of work you do than on the exact kind of food that you eat.

No one nation has a monopoly of "Strong Men." In East India there are "Strong Men" by the dozen, and most of these Hindus live on rice and highly spiced meat dishes. I have seen giant Chinamen who ate nothing but rice. I have seen enormously powerful Scandinavians who seemed to live entirely on fish. There are in the north of Italy some very strong men whose staple diet is macaroni, boiled chestnuts and white bread. I know personally some amateur "Strong Men" in New England who eat almost nothing except pork and beans. I can show you negroes and mulattoes who are magnificently built and very, very strong; if given a choice, they will live entirely on chicken and pork chops. Going to the opposite extreme, there are famous Turkish "Strong Men" who would rather die than eat one mouthful of pork.

Super-strength is a matter of bodily proportions and muscular strength, and I am convinced that you can get such proportions and such strength, no matter what kind of food you eat, so long as you do the right kind of muscular work.

I am perfectly well aware that there are many people who have no desire to become very strong, although many of them wish to become bigger and better built. To such people it seems a great deal easier to add to the size of the body by eating a certain kind of food than by doing any kind of work. When I first became interested in the subject of strength, most of the lifting records were held by Germans, and the popular idea was that the

184

Germans got their strength by drinking beer. Some of their athletes were enormously powerful just because they are so big and heavy. In the last few years it has been proven that a finely developed man of moderate weight can lift just about as much as the biggest and fattest giant of the beer-drinking type.

I believe that a man who takes up bar-bell exercise should drink plenty of sweet milk; eat meat at least once a day; eggs at least once a day, and such vegetables and fruits as tempt his appetite. I can see no reason why one should eat bran, or whole wheat, or cereals, in place of white bread. I believe that a man will get the most benefit out of foods that he likes, and that it is a mistake to adopt a diet composed of distasteful foods. It seems to me impossible that a man can make any great improvement by eating a limited quantity of foods which are so distasteful that he gets no enjoyment from his meals.

Providing that you do the right kind of exercise and satisfy your appetite, you can eat almost anything. I know one celebrated "Strong Man" who eats ice-cream three times a day, and several plates of it at each meal. The late Arthur Saxon, who was certainly one of the strongest men of our time, used to consume an average of four dozen bottles of beer every day.

The only restriction in regards to your diet is that you should indulge only moderately in candy and pastry; but after you have trained for a while you will find that you desire solid foods, and that chocolate and pie will lose their appeal.

One time I was visited by a "Strong Man" from the Middle West. He took part in one of our lifting carnivals and created one world's record on that visit. The day after the exhibition we went out to lunch together and he ordered a beefsteak. The waiter brought him a steak about four inches square and nearly two inches thick. Along with it he had three glasses of milk, and he finished up with a dish of rice pudding. When he was through he said, "You know, Mr. Calvert, we can't get meat like this where I come from. If you keep me here a month and see that I can get a steak like that every day, I'll break every record that was ever made." He claimed that he felt much stronger after eating beefsteak than after eating a meal composed entirely of bread and vegetables.

Most "Strong Men" are very deliberate eaters. They chew their food very thoroughly, and sometimes I wonder whether their habit of thorough mastication is not responsible for a large part of their strength. Most men who use bar-bells develop very powerful jaws, and most of them have very good teeth. The strength of the jaw seems to be entirely a by-product of the bodily exercise, because very few of these men ever do the so-called "iron- jaw" lifting. In the same way, their necks get thicker and rounder, even if they do not specialize on neck exercises. If a man has a 44-inch chest, his neck should measure about 16½ inches; and it seems to be true that if a man increases his chest from 36 to 44 inches, his neck, which measured 14 inches at the start, will grow to measure 15½ inches, even if he never does any "wrestler's bridge" work. Strength of neck and strength of jaw seem to go together. The size and shape of your neck is an indication of your vitality; and it is commonly accepted that a man with a powerful, square jaw has more vital force than a man with a small and weak jaw. It is not necessary to do any special work to develop your jaw, outside of thoroughly chewing the food.

Every once in a while you come across some exception which seems to destroy the value of a rule. Most of us believe that a good set of teeth is about as valuable a possession as a man can have. It seems perfectly reasonable to say that without a good set of teeth a man could not become strong. It seems equally reasonable to say that if a man or boy ate candy to excess he would become soft and flabby. A number of years ago a young

186

man of eighteen became seized with the ambition to become very strong, and started training with bar-bells. This youth's mother had kept a candy shop, and when a small boy he had put in his spare time eating candy. When I first knew him all his teeth were in bad condition, and the six teeth in the center of the upper-jaw had rotted to such an extent that there were only stumps left. I give you my word that inside of a year's time that young man had gained enormously in strength and had become famous for the beauty of his figure. Later on, he made some amateur lifting- records ; and still later, some of our best-known sculptors employed him as a model. All of them raved about his build and wondered at his strength. After all this, when he was about to go on the professional stage, he had the stumps of his teeth extracted and now wears a plate. This sort of case is very upsetting to one's pet ideas and theories. One would have thought that a youth who had lost some of his teeth at the age of fourteen, and whose system must have been overloaded with saccharine, would thereby be prevented from making any noticeable improvement. When he took up bar-bell exercise he stopped eating candy, but he did not make any other change in his diet. It must have been the kind of exercise he took which so improved his figure and increased his development. If I had not seen the thing happen, I would hardly have believed it.

On any big athletic team, the sprinters and the long distance runners have to train vigorously, and their diet is carefully supervised; but the big weight-throwers train very little, and eat and drink anything they feel like. All they have to do is to practice at their particular lift; that is, "put-the-shot" and "throw-the-hammer" or the "56-pound weight." If you wish to become super-strong, and are willing to take the exercise, and are careful to satisfy your appetite, you do not have to bother any more about your diet than do these big weight-throwers.

The truth of the matter is, that as a man develops super- strength in his muscles, his internal organs acquire much greater vigor. Perhaps I have stated the case backwards. It may be that the improvement in the functional power of the organs takes place before the muscles grow in size and strength. Undoubtedly, the muscles would not grow so rapidly unless they were continually supplied with fresh material from the blood. The quality of the blood is dependent on the perfect working of the digestive and assimilative organs, and these organs seem to be stimulated and invigorated by vigorous exercise. Thin, anaemic individuals are said to have a "weak stomach," and no person with a weak stomach can be fundamentally strong. I believe that organs can be strong or weak just as the exterior muscles can be likewise; also that it is possible to strengthen the organs to the same degree to which you can strengthen the exterior muscles.

When you use the expression, "a week stomach," you do not mean that the material composing the wall of the stomach is weak, but that the stomach functions feebly; that is, it does not secrete the digestive juices, nor do its part in digesting the food. A man with a "weak stomach" is easily upset by a couple of glasses of liquor, and is apt to become nauseated either by overeating or by partaking of certain kinds of food. A man with a very strong stomach is one who can digest anything, and whose digestive functions are so perfect that he can quickly and thoroughly assimilate anything he puts in his stomach. Such a man can consume a very large quantity of liquor without showing the slightest signs of intoxication. Likewise, if he eats a large quantity of very rich foods, his stomach acts so perfectly that the food is thoroughly digested and there are no after-effects.

Mr. John L. Sullivan, besides being the champion fighter of his time, was physically one of the strongest men in the world. As a youth, he was a bar-bell lifter and traveled under the name "the Boston Strong Boy." Undoubtedly, his early training with bar-bells had a great deal to do with his tremendous muscular strength, and with the almost unequaled vigor of his digestion. It is related that on one occasion, Sullivan won a bet by consuming one hundred mixed drinks in the course of one evening without becoming intoxicated.

Now please do not think that I am suggesting that drinking is the proper thing for a "Strong Man." Sullivan died before he was 60 years old. A few years before his death, he became a violent prohibitionist. If he had used liquor in moderation, he probably would have lived to be ninety. Arthur Saxon's continual and inordinate drinking of beer may have weakened his constitution; although it is said that Saxon's death at the age of forty- eight was due partly to the injuries he had sustained in the War. Beer-drinking is supposed to make one stout: but Saxon never showed any surplus flesh, although it was not an infrequent thing for him to drink as many as one hundred glasses of beer in one day.

Besides having a strong stomach, a man of super-strength must be possessed of great vigor in the other assimilative organs, and he must have a sound solid heart and large, high-quality lungs.

It would be the height of folly to exercise just for the sake of getting big muscles on the outside of one's body. Strength comes from within. The saving fact is that in order to get big muscles, it is necessary to have a vigorous digestive system, and in order to fully develop the strength of the muscles, it is necessary to have a sound nervous system, sound heart and powerful lungs. Any system of training worthy of the name strengthens the inside of the body, as well as the outside of the body.

I have seen men with weak stomachs, poor digestions and low nervous force so change themselves by properly graded progressive exercise, that in the course of a few months they acquired the digestion of an ostrich, great nervous force and, at the same time, increased their bodily weight thirty or forty pounds; and that weight was all good, solid, muscular tissue. I have seen fat men start with a 40-inch chest measurement and a 48-inch waist measurement, and without dieting increase the chest measurement to 44 inches and reduce the waist to 34 inches; and, what is more, I have seen these men hold their gains for years and never relapse into being very fat or very thin, even after they discontinued their exercise.

A workman who spends eight hours a day using a pick and shovel, or a lumberman who swings an ax and carries heavy logs for the same amount of time, can, and does, eat an amount and a variety of food which a slender, indoor worker would find impossible to digest. It should be remembered that a workman is continually leaning over, both directly forwards and to the side, and that he is continually using the muscles of the loins, the sides of the waist, and the front of the abdomen. Those muscles form the wall of the lower body and enclose the digestive organs. Every time you bend over and pick up a weight, whether it is one end of a log, a shovelful of dirt, or a 50-lb. bar-bell you call into vigorous action those muscles of the waist region. The continued bending massages, compresses and shakes up the digestive organs, and the continued work develops the muscles in the neighborhood of the organs. A large, well-developed muscle draws more blood to it than does a small, undeveloped muscle. Men who have a fine set of muscles around the waist never suffer from digestive troubles. Such common ailments as "gas on the stomach" (flatulence), and constipation can be permanently banished by developing the muscles around your waist. As you develop the "washboard pattern" of muscles on the front of the abdomen and stomach, the intestines will become able to do more and better work. While you are developing the muscles on the small of the back and those at the sides of the waist, you're adding to the tone of your liver. Such exercises as those shown

190

in Figs. 32 and 33 are much more effective in curing constipation than shaking up the liver by horseback riding.

The exercises which strengthen the muscles which lie across the loins and near the lower part of the spine greatly augment virility. This is a subject which cannot be discussed in this book, but any user of bar-bells can tell you that remarkable increase in vigor comes from developing the lower part of the back.

Men who are thin and undeveloped really suffer from some form of malnutrition; that is, the assimilative organs fail to draw the proper nutrition from the food, and that means that the blood quality is poor.

Most excessively stout men are in that condition simply because they neglect to use the muscles of the waist, although it is true that some men are fat because of the improper working of some gland. The ordinary stout man can reduce his waist by the same exercises which build up the figure of the thin man. Fat cannot exist in, or near, an active muscle. That explains why some stout men have slender arms and slender calves long after the rest of the body has become hung with fat. The forearms and calves of the legs are the only parts of the body which they use continually.

In conclusion, I wish to say emphatically that in order to be super-strong a man has to be super-healthy. If you train properly, so as to increase the vigor of your internal organs at the same time that you are increasing the exterior development, you will get the kind of muscle that will stay with you the rest of your life, and you can create an upright, shapely figure that will not become bowed and enfeebled until extreme old age.

CHAPTER XIX

MUSCLE CONTROL

The strength of a muscle is its ability to contract against great resistance. Strength is partly a matter of will-power, that is, of mental control over the muscles. Just the same, no man can make himself strong just by an effort of the will. The size of a muscle has a great deal to do with its strength. If there are two men of exactly equal measurements, the one who has the great amount of will power, or mental control over his muscles, will be the stronger of the two. Nevertheless, no slender, small-muscled man, no matter how great his mental control over his muscles, can hope to equal the strength of a man whose muscles are twice as big, and who has an equal control over them.

There is a great deal of unnecessary mystery about this subject of "muscle control." It is one of the simplest things in the world. You have been exercising a while, and your arms have gotten considerably bigger and much more muscular than formerly. If you get into a discussion concerning muscular development you are apt to say to your opponent, "Well, feel my arm!" And as he puts his hand on your upper arm you bend your arm at right angles, and tighten the muscles of the upper arm so as to make it bigger and harder. That is "muscle control." Anyone can do it. If you will think back you will recall that every time you ask a friend to feel your arm you instinctively bend the arm at right angles, so as to put the muscles in a favorable position for contraction. If you are a beginner you are apt to bend your arm all the way, so as to make the biceps muscles stick up in a large hump; but if you are experienced you know that if you bend the arm only at right angles it is possible for you to harden the biceps on the front of the upper arm and, at the same time, harden the triceps on the back of the upper arm; thus making your arm bigger than if you flexed and hardened only the biceps muscle.

For many years it was a custom for a professional "Strong Man" to open his act by doing a few minutes' "muscle-posing" in a lighted cabinet. Such cabinets were usually made of a dark material, so as to make a contrast with the flesh of the athlete. At the top of the cabinet and out of sight of the audience were one or more very powerful lights, with reflectors so arranged that they threw a strong downward illumination on the body of the athlete. This strong light from above accentuated the shadows thrown by the muscles. In some cabinets it was possible to switch off the top light and turn on a light placed at the height of the athlete's elbow; and this light would throw shadows sidewise, and would bring out details of development which would not be revealed by a high light. The "Strong Man," standing on a low pedestal in the middle of the cabinet would strike one attitude after another, thereby displaying to the greatest advantage the prodigious development of his muscles. If you were so lucky as to see several different men pose you would notice that they all employed the same positions; that in order to show the biceps muscles to best advantage they would hold the arms in a certain position; that to show the abdominal muscles fully flexed they would bend their bodies in a certain way. 'There is a fixed routine of such positions or movements which is known to every professional and most amateur "Strong Men," and if you learn the positions and have sufficient development you can make a most amazing display, because as you go from one position to another different sets of muscles will be flexed, and huge bands and masses of muscle will appear on different parts of your body. The average reporter in describing such an act will say that the athlete's muscles moved about under his skin "like a mass of snakes writhing under a blanket."

All this posing work is simply a matter of "muscle control." The fundamental principle of "muscle control" is, that before you can flex or contract a muscle to its fullest extent you must place the body or the limb in the most favorable position. For instance, if you hold your elbow at your side and double up the right arm you can make the biceps muscle very hard, but that muscle will not be fully flexed. If you put the right hand behind your neck, and raise your right elbow as high as you can, as in Fig. 91, you can flex the biceps muscle with much greater force, and it will be bigger than it is when the elbow is at the side of the waist. If you wish to get full control of your biceps you have to first raise your arm in this position. After the elbow is up, harden the biceps as much as you can. Then release the tension and your biceps muscle will become softer and the humped-up appearance will disappear. If you keep your elbow up, and flex and relax the biceps several times in succession, you will find that after a couple of weeks' practice you can make the biceps stand up in a much more impressive curve than it formerly did.

When you have your elbow up, as in Fig. 91, you will find it impossible to harden the triceps muscle on the back of the upper arm, because that muscle has been stretched by bending the arm at the elbow. In order to get control of your triceps you have to stand with the hands clasped behind the hips, as in Fig. 92. In that position, if you press the elbows towards the back and press the hands outward, the triceps muscles will flex themselves, as shown in the picture. The moment you relax the tension the triceps muscles will relax and the back of the arm becomes perfectly smooth.

That shows you the general principle of "muscle control." It is easiest for most physical culturists to control the upper-arm muscles, because most of their developing work has been devoted to the cultivation of those muscles; but when he tries to do the same thing with the muscles of his back, his chest, his abdomen and his legs he can't make nearly as good a display; because, in the first place, he does not know the positions most favorable to contraction (and therefore, for display); and in the second place his muscles are not big enough to be impressive

194

even if he does learn how to contract them. Most of the large muscles on the body and the limbs can be brought under mental control just as easily as can the arm muscles.

Fig. 93 shows an athlete with remarkably developed chest muscles. In this picture those muscles are relaxed, in fact, the whole body is relaxed, and this man's breast muscles are so large that they sag slightly of their own weight. Fig. 94 shows the same athlete with all his muscles flexed. You can hardly believe it is the same man, and the immense difference in his appearance is caused by an alteration in position and by "muscle control." The muscles on the breast bring the arms forward. In Fig. 94 the athlete is pressing his hands against each other with great force, and this has flexed the breast muscles and entirely altered their outlines. At the same time he has hardened the muscles on the shoulders, the arms and on the front of the abdomen. The beginner has to be satisfied with flexing one or two muscles at a time; but a bar-bell user, like this man, can instantly and simultaneously flex every muscle in the body. If you want to get control of your breast muscles you can do so by assuming the position shown in Fig. 94 and pressing the palms of the hands against each other. After a while you will get so that you can stand in a perfectly normal position and simply by thinking about it, harden the muscles on the breast and completely alter their outlines. But (and this is a very big "but") the flexed muscles will not look like much unless you have already made them big and thick by proper exercise. I have been familiar with this subject of "muscle control" for over thirty years. In 1893 I saw Eugen Sandow do most of the feats of "muscle control" that have since been done by other athletes. When Sandow was standing or sitting at ease his body and limbs, while of great size, were just as smooth as those of a Greek statue, although by a mere effort of the will he could make muscles stand out in knots and ridges all over him. Any other bar-bell user can do the same thing. After you get your muscles by work you can do marvels in the

195

way of "muscle control"; but you cannot develop strong muscles or big muscles by simply flexing and relaxing them through an effort of the will.

The best exponents of "muscle control" are former bar-bell users. The man who is best known as an exponent of "muscle control" was making lifting records several years before he advocated "muscle control" as a means of development. As far as I can see his muscles were just as big and just as much under his control when he was doing bar-bell work exclusively as they are today. Perhaps the most skillful man in this line is a lifter by the name of Nowielsky, who is known on the stage as Otto Arco. Figs. 95 and 96 show two of his "muscle control" stunts. In Fig. 95 he is showing the rope of muscles on the abdomen at the same time that he displays the muscles of his arms and shoulders. (By the way, he is the originator of this "isolated control" of the abdominal muscles.) Fig. 96 shows what looks like an incredible development of the muscles on the upper back, but part of the effect is obtained by his control over his shoulder blades. In this pose, by flexing certain muscles, he has spread the shoulder blades apart and changed the angle at which they are usually inclined. I give you my word that when this man is standing at a normal position, with his arms hanging at his sides, his back does not show these extraordinary contours. His back is very broad and packed from shoulder to shoulder with wonderfully developed muscles, but when he is not flexing those muscles, the back, while perfectly shaped, is not humped up with muscle. But when he raises his arm in the position shown, spreads his shoulder blades and flexes all the muscles on the upper back, he looks just as in Fig. 96. It is quite possible for you to learn to spread your shoulder blades just as he has done, and you may make your flexed muscles just as hard as his are when flexed; but unless your muscles are fully developed you will not be able to duplicate the effect of his pose.

Sandow used to say that, while on an exhibition tour, he never deliberately exercised. He claimed that the two exhibitions he gave every day afforded him plenty of hard muscular work, and that in between times he could keep his muscles in condition just by "flicking" them while sitting in a chair reading his newspaper. By "flicking" them he meant alternately flexing and relaxing them. I believe it is true that after you have developed your muscles you can keep them close to the highest pitch of development by practicing "muscle control" for a few minutes a day; but your muscles will not grow any bigger or stronger.

"Muscle control" is all right as a means of displaying your muscles, but it positively is not a source of increased strength or development. I have seen skinny men practice "muscle control" stunts for months without adding one inch to the size of the chest, or as much as a quarter of an inch to the size of the arms or legs. True, they were able to make such muscles as they had stand out in knots. Anyone can do that if he can learn the correct positions. Your little brother can learn to control his biceps muscle by putting his arm in the position described in the first part of this chapter, but after he does flex the muscle it is just one tiny lump. On the other hand, if you, personally have big arms, a little practice in the proper positions will enable you to display your muscles to far better advantage than if you did not know these positions. In Fig. 97 you see what looks like two immense lumps of muscle projecting from each side of the upper back. If you stretch your arms straight above your head, as this man is doing, and then after the arms are straight, reach as high as you can with your hands, thus lifting the shoulders, your shoulder blades will spread apart. If you shoulder blades are covered with big, powerfully developed muscles you will look just as this man does; but if you have very little muscle on the upper back, although the edges of the shoulder blades will push the skin outward, your back will not look like the back in this picture. Before you can make any great muscular display through "muscle control" you must have the muscle to start with. The bigger and stronger your muscles are, the more you can do in the way of controlling and displaying them.

(Referring back to Fig. 95 we see the one exception to the general rule. The ordinary athlete, when he wishes to play the abdominal muscles, leans slightly forward and contracts those muscles so that they appear in horizontal ridges, as in Fig. 34. This man, Arco, accidentally discovered that if the lungs were almost emptied of air there would be a partial vacuum created, and that when you flexed the front abdominal muscles the sides of the abdomen would cave in, as in the picture.) I consider that "muscle control" is valuable as a supplementary exercise, and that it is invaluable to the athlete who wishes to do muscular posing. Almost any exercise is good. Even "muscle control" has some value, because if you go through all the different positions which display all the different muscles in the body you get at least a little exercise out of it.

There are some other details which may interest you. If you can control your muscles you can, in certain poses, produce some very pleasing effects. In Fig. 98 the athlete's back is very broad at the line of the arm pits and comparatively narrow at the waist. He had made his back broad by spreading his shoulders apart; but it should be noted that as he does spread the shoulders the muscles in the middle of the back seem to disappear. That man can deliberately press his shoulder blades together and make his back nearly six inches narrower than in this pose, and when he does bring his shoulder blades together the middle of the upper back is covered with mounds of muscle. If he stands up in this position, and first spreads his shoulders and then squeezes them together, and repeats the motion a dozen times he is getting some valuable exercise for those muscles in the upper back which control these two motions. But again, the reason he can make himself so extraordinarily broad is because in the first place he has a big rib box, and in the second place his upper-back muscles are unusually big and powerful. If you can induce some thin man to try this stunt you will find that by pressing his shoulders together, then spreading them apart, the width of his back will be altered only an inch or so (that is, when he spreads his shoulders his back is only an inch wider than when he squeezes them together). If you are lucky enough to get hold of an amateur "Strong Man" and bar-bell user (one of these chaps with a 44-inch normal chest) you will find that he can make a difference of 6 inches in the width of his back, according to how he holds his shoulders. The star of this stunt was Joe Nordquest. Fig. 99 shows his extraordinary ability to voluntarily broaden his upper back. You must remember that Nordquest's chest measures 46 inches normal, and that his upper arm measures nearly 18 inches. So if your chest measures only 36 and your arms only 13 inches, you must not expect to duplicate the effect that he gets.

Most advocates of "muscle control" confine their practice entirely to the arm muscles and the abdominal muscles; whereas they could get very good all-around exercise if they devoted part of their time to getting control of the muscles on their back, their sides and their legs. If you stand squarely on both feet and then lock your knees back, you can harden the muscles on the front and outside of the thighs. If your thighs are of a fair size when you harden the muscles the thighs will assume the shape shown in Fig. 91; but if your thighs are thin, you can harden the muscles but the shape of the thighs will hardly be altered at all. The bigger and more powerfully developed the thighs are the more you can do in the way of mentally controlling your muscles. Mr. Max Unger, when doing cabinet-posing, could do more with his thigh muscles than any other man I have seen; that is, he could flex the thigh muscles in different ways, make them apparently jump up and down, and also move them from side to side without the slightest movement of the limbs themselves. He would stand squarely on both feet and make his thigh muscles move in a most extraordinary way, so that it seemed as though the muscles were being flexed by some outside power; whereas it was entirely a matter of muscular control. If Mr. Unger's thighs had been thin the movements of the muscles would hardly have been perceptible; but his thighs were of extraordinary size and power and beautifully shaped.

It would take too much space to describe the several dozen positions which you must learn if you wish to get complete mental control of all the muscles in the body; but if you will observe the rule that you must first put yourself in a position that causes one muscle to contract, it is then easy to get control of that muscle. Some of you may have trouble in hardening the muscles on the front of your thigh when standing erect; although most of you will be able to do so if you make your legs perfectly straight and push the knees as far back as possible. If, however, you stand in front of a chair and raise the right leg and place the heel on the seat of the chair with your leg straight, you will find it very easy to harden the muscles on the front of the thigh. This is because one function of those muscles is to raise the leg forward. Similarly, if you want to get control of the muscle at the right side of the waist, you must bend the body over to the right, which contracts that muscle.

After a few weeks' practice you will find that you can flex many of the muscles on the body without the necessity of bending the body from side to side. While seated in a chair you can, by a simple effort of the will, flex the breast muscles, or you can just as easily flex the big muscles on the upper back which lie close to the arm pit. You will be able to temporarily change the shape of your upper back through your control of the muscles which move the shoulder blades; but you must remember that it is far easier to learn mental control of a well-developed muscle than of one which is thin and undeveloped.

I believe that one reason why bar-bell users have such "muscle control" is that their practice of lifting has developed extreme speed. This statement will come as a revelation to some of you who think that weight-lifting stiffens a man's muscles and makes him slow in action. That may have been true of the old-time lifter; but the modern lifter has to be as quick as a boxer with his hands and with his feet. In making what we call the "quick lifts," the lifter has to learn to entirely change his position in a fraction of a second. This would be impossible unless his muscles responded instantaneously to the message telegraphed from the brain through the motor nerves and to the muscles themselves.

Recently I had occasion to take some photographs to illustrate some details of lifting. I had only an hour in which to get a model. The photographer happened to know of a hand-balancer who in his youth had gotten a fine development by using bar-bells. We telephoned the man and asked him if he was in shape to pose. He replied that although he had retired from the stage, and that it had been twelve years since he had seen a bar-bell, nevertheless, he was in perfect shape. A few minutes later he reported for the job, and stripped so that we could see his development. In order to prove that he was in condition he held up his right arm with the elbow slightly bent. There was not the least tension of the muscles of his upper arm, and the upper edge of the arm was perfectly smooth. He quickly flexed his muscles and his biceps simply leaped into a high curve. He did this several times in succession, contracting and releasing the muscles with such speed that the eye could hardly follow the movements of the muscles. When the upper arm is held out to the side and the muscles relaxed, the large muscles will sag a trifle of their own weight, so that most of the muscle seems to be below the bone. That was the way this man's arm appeared before he flexed his muscles; but when he did flex his biceps the lower edge of the arm became taut, and the upper edge (the biceps) mounted in so high a curve that his arm was apparently two inches thicker than before. This man had never even heard the phrase "muscle control"; but the bar-bell training which he had done in his youth had given him a development which he had never lost, and a mental control over his muscles which he still retains, and which enables him to still flex any muscle in his body simply by concentrating his mind on it.

I don't want you to take my word for all this,—I would like you to try it. If you have no development you will be sadly disappointed by your efforts at "muscle control"; but if you have big and powerful muscles developed either through the use of bar-bells or other kinds of vigorous exercise, you will find that in a few weeks you will be able to do almost any stunt of "muscle control" that you have seen in a picture, or actually done by a "Strong Man."

I have, at various times, been paid visits by lifters and bar-bell users who were interested in the subject of "muscle control," and invariably, in the course of half an hour, I have been able to show them how to learn to control their muscles. Those men already had the development and the mental control, and all I had to do v/as to show them the positions. On the contrary, I have never been able to do this with an undeveloped man, because such a man is handicapped by the fact that he has no muscle to speak of, and cannot control what little muscle he has. "Muscle control" is a thing that comes to you while you are developing the muscles; but it will not create muscular tissue nor will it make you any bigger or stronger.

PLATE 63

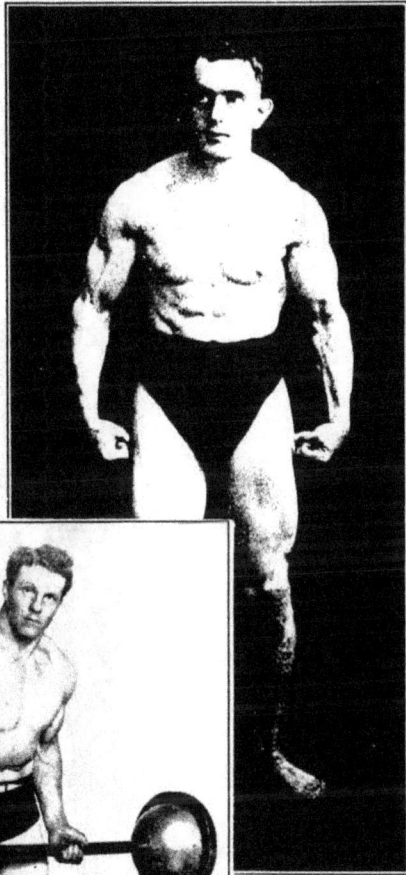

Fig. 131

Figure 131 (above). Robert Dallas, an amateur lifter who has a magnificent chest and shoulder development

Fig. 130

Plate 63, Figure 130 (below). Henry Steinborn doing a two-arm "Curl" with 173 lbs., a feat which he repeated six times in succession

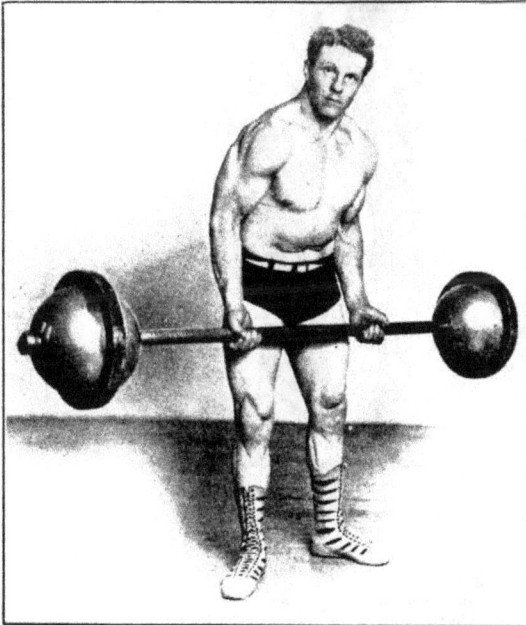

PLATE 64

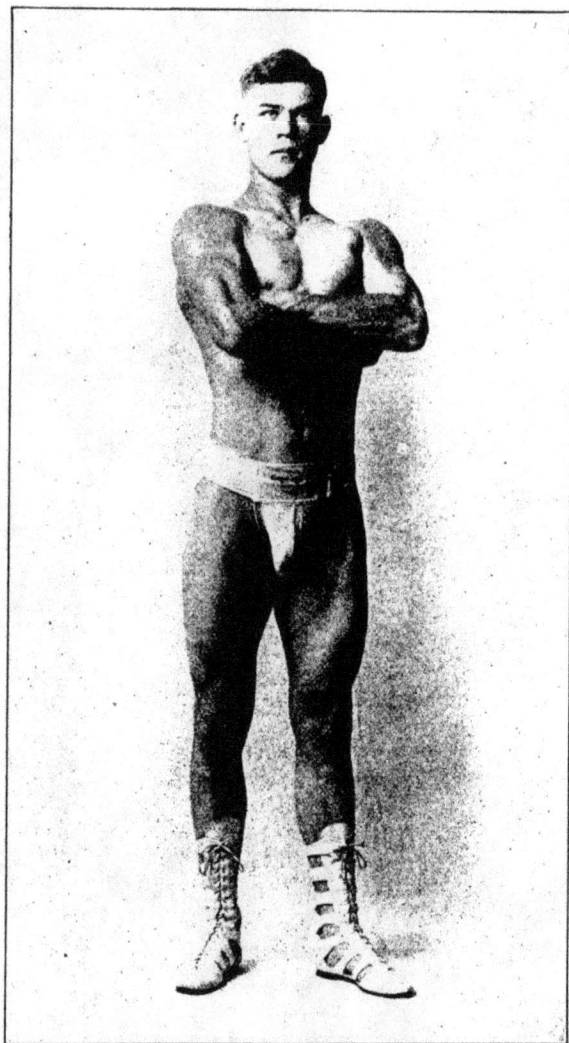

Fig. 132

Plate 64, Figure 132. Harry B. Paschall, who got his development through the medium of bar-bell exercise. He is
a light-boned man of the Apollo type.

PLATE 65

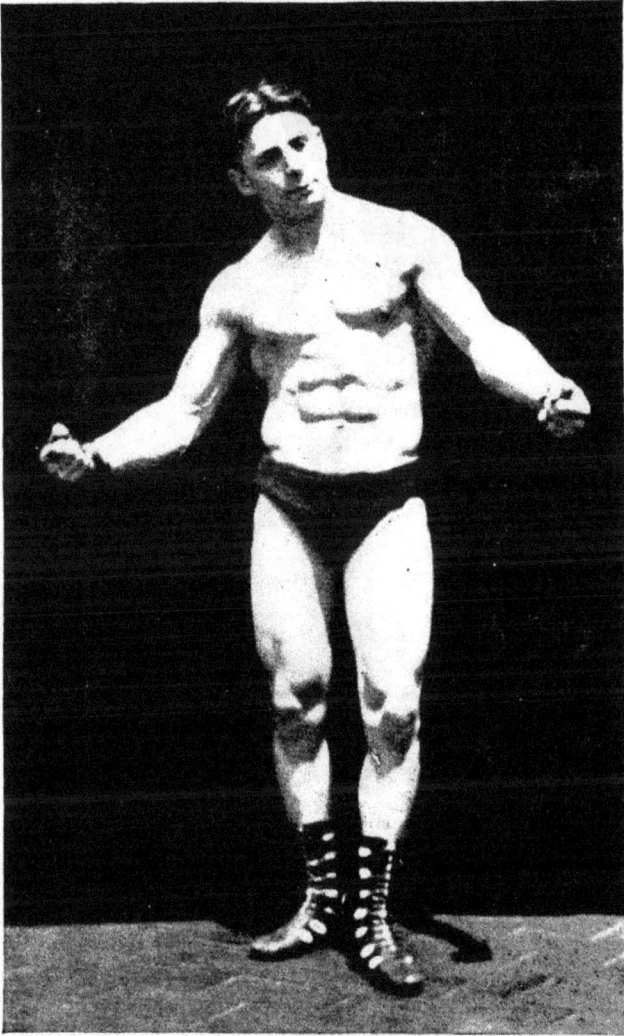

Fig. 133

Plate 65, Figure 133. Sigmund Klein, whose bodily proportions
are almost perfect, and who is probably the best developed of
the younger generation of lifters

PLATE 66

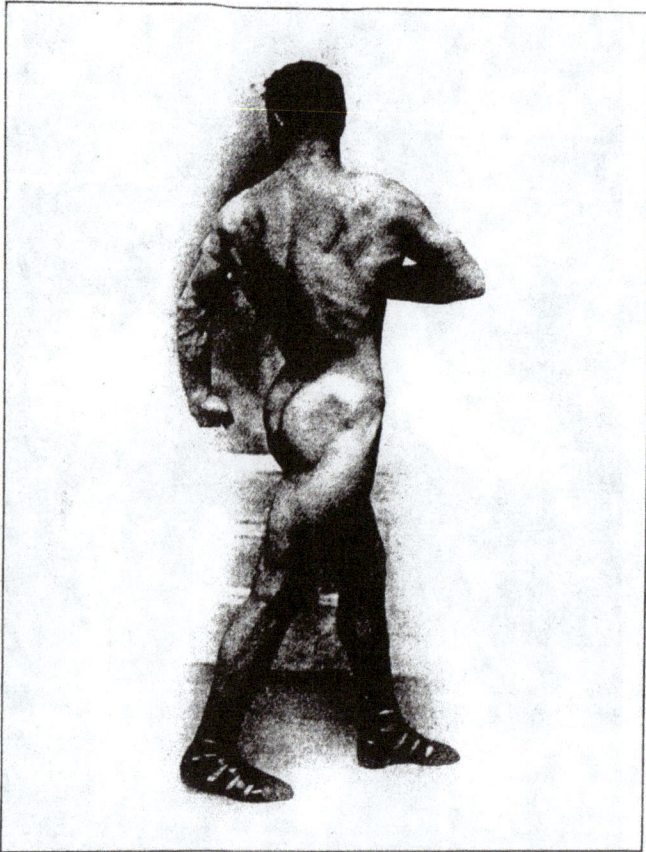

Fig. 134

Plate 66, Figure 134. Matysek in a pose which displays the great
breadth of his shoulders and back. You cannot duplicate this
pose unless you are very flexible, as well as highly developed.
This effect is gained by twisting the body until the shoulders are
at right angles to the hips

PLATE 67

Fig. 135

Plate 67, Figure
135 (above). Alex-
ander Karasick, an
amateur, who has a
chest like Hacken-
schmidt's.

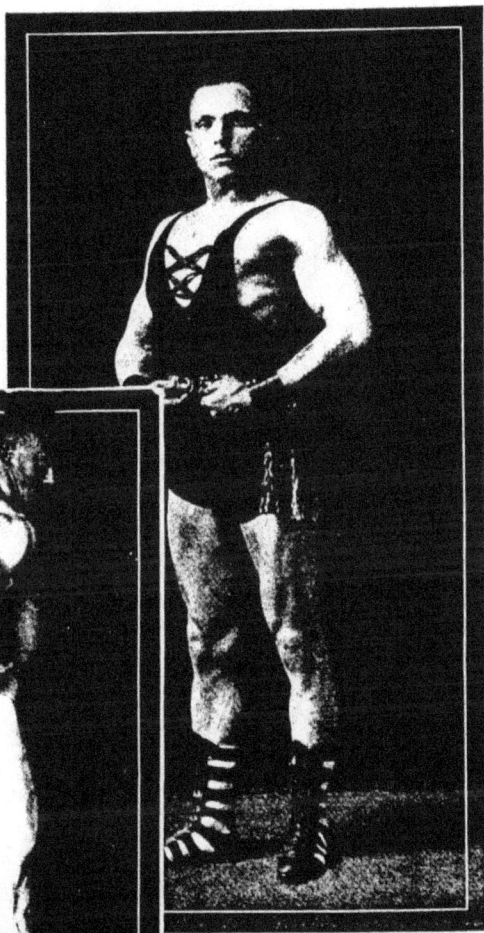

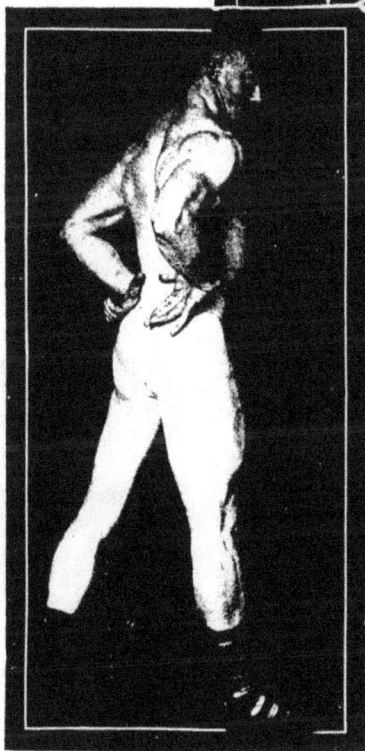

Fig. 136

Figure 136 (below). Owen Carr
in an extremely effective pose,
which shows his magnificent proportions, as well as his wonderful
development.

207

PLATE 68

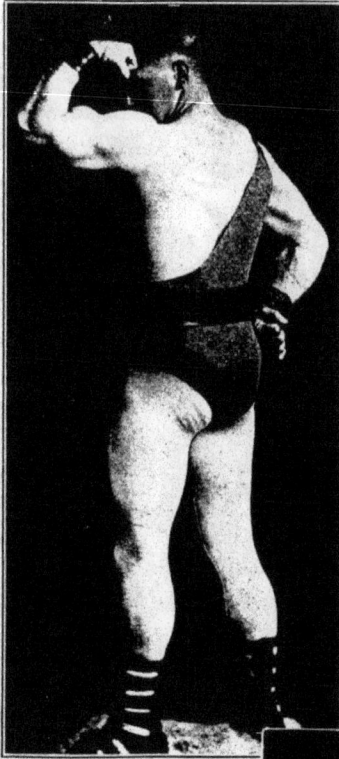

Fig. 137

Plate 68, Figure 137 (above).
Ig. Neubauer, who became
famous as "The Strong Man
of the Navy." An interesting pose, because it shows
the forearms from two different points of view. Notice
how he has bulked up his
right forearm by clinching
the fist, and then bending the
wrist inward. The splendid
development of the legs adds
to the impression of power

Fig. 138

Figure 138 (below).
An unusual Kodak pic-
ture, showing Sigmund
Klein in a pose which
displays his arm and
upper body muscles to
the greatest advantage

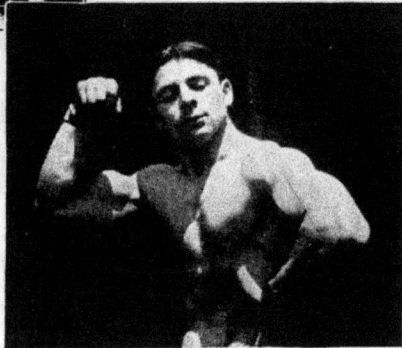

PLATE 69

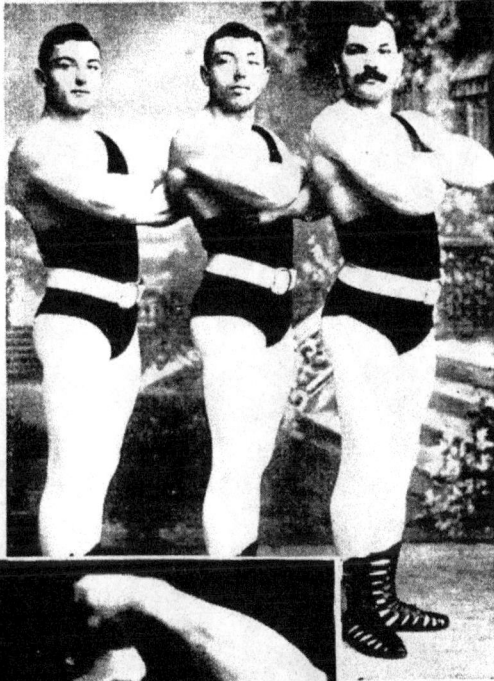

Fig. 139

Plate 69, Figure 139 (below). The famous Arthur Saxon. Although Saxon's measurements were bigger than Sandow's, his muscular development was not as noticeable, because his bones, and therefore his joints were larger. He could have made his left forearm look better if he had followed the example of Neubauer, as in Figure 137

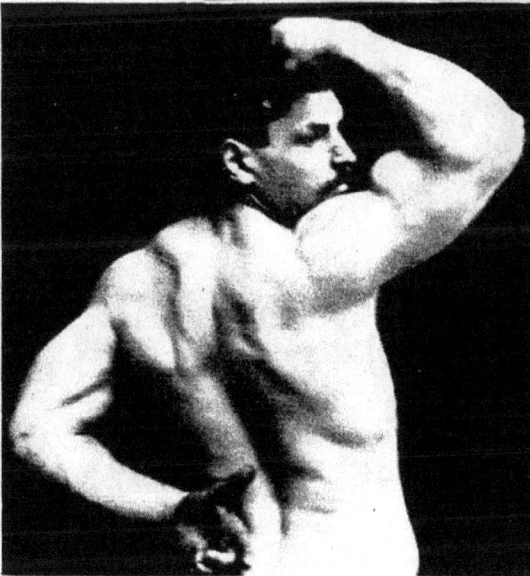

Fig. 140

Figure 140 (above). The Saxon trio. At the right, Arthur (Otto), the oldest brother; in the center Kurt, the youngest; and at the left, Herman, the most beautifully built of the three

PLATE 70

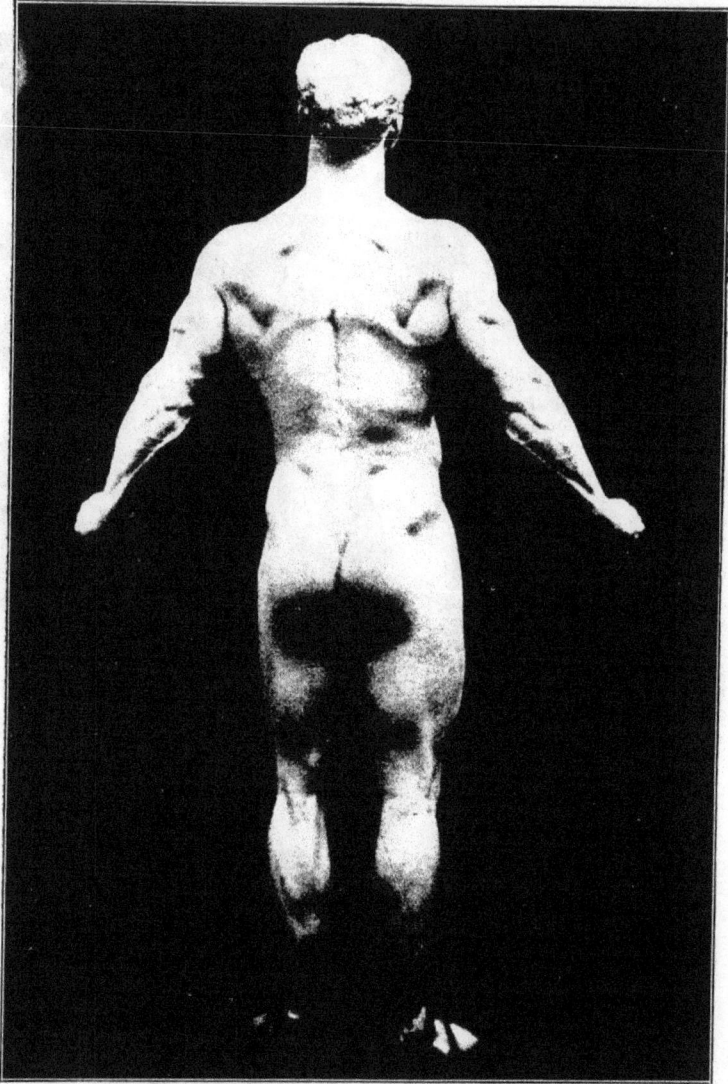

Fig. 141

Plate 70, Figure 141. Adolph Nordquest, whose figure so resembles Sandow's that the two were often mistaken for brothers

CHAPTER XX

PROFESSIONAL EXHIBITION WORK

The average citizen rarely sees a heavy bar-bell except when it is being used on the stage by some vaudeville "Strong Man." Consequently Mr. Average Citizen gets the idea that if he used a bar-bell he would have to do the same enormous lifts which are customarily shown in "Strong" acts.

The exhibition stunts you see performed by professional "Strong Men" have very little to do with the creation of strength. The professional does his training before he goes on the stage. For every one professional who does exhibition work, there are a thousand men and boys who use adjustable bar-bells for the purpose of improving their bodies. There are a great number of amateur lifters; but all these amateurs have put in several months at bodybuilding exercises with their bar-bells before they start the practice of actual lifting. I have never known a man to start training with the idea of becoming a professional, although I know several amateurs who have become so enormously strong that they have been induced by theatrical managers to appear professionally. If you train with bar-bells, you are not compelled to do any real lifting. If your aim is to become beautifully built and enormously strong, you can achieve your ambition just by practicing the developing exercises described in this book.

That part of the public which patronizes the theaters has very little interest in bar-bell and dumbbell lifting. They enjoy seeing "Strong acts"; but their preference is for marvelous and seemingly miraculous feats of strength. Therefore, professional lifters cater to the taste of their audiences. Instead of lifting bar-bells, they lift and support enormous quantities of live and dead weight. They try to make their acts spectacular.

After you have practiced for a while with bar-bells, you discover some very surprising things. For example, you find that while it is difficult to "push up" to arms' length a 15 bar-bell, that it requires but little exertion to hold the bell a once you have straightened your arm. Every professional is fully aware of this fact, and it is quite natural that they should take advantage of their knowledge. In Fig. 100, you see a picture of a man walking while holding a bar-bell at arms' length. In doing this stunt he keeps his arm locked straight so that the forearm and upper arm are in one line. He walks with his knees slightly bent. Almost all the work is done by the thighs. If he arched his back and had his arm bent at the elbow he would find great difficulty in walking with the bell, but by keeping his arm and back in one straight line and walking with bent knees the feat becomes trivial. George Lurich, in his performance, used to walk across the stage while supporting five men with his upraised right arm. Fig. 101 shows Anton Matysek walking with a bicycle and three men—a total weight of about 500 lbs. Eugen Sandow used to carry a small horse at arms' length. The horse was hauled in the air by means of a block and tackle. Sandow would stoop under the horse and grab hold of a loop on the side of a girth which passed around the horse's body. In performing this stunt, Sandow would lean forward and allow some of the horse's weight to rest on his shoulders. In Fig. 101 Matysek has bent slightly forward from the hips so that the lower part of the bicycle-frame rests against his back. Matysek could "push up" 250 lbs. with one arm; but he could carry 600 lbs. on the straight arm. Sandow could "push up" 271 lbs., and the horse he carried must have weighed at least 800 lbs. Sandow himself stated that after his arm was straight, he could carry almost any weight.

I believe stunts like this to be entirely legitimate in stage work. If a man comes out and pushes up a 200-lb. bar-bell the onlookers are not very much impressed; because, to tell the truth, they do not know whether the record is 200 lbs. or 300 lbs.; but the audience gets very enthusiastic when a man comes out and carries on his straight arm several hundred pounds of live weight, like the three men on Matysek's bicycle or like Sandow's horse.

Another well-known exhibition stunt is the one illustrated in Fig. 102. After the athlete gets into the "bridge" position, an attendant places on his shoulders and knees the lower of the two planks. The upper plank, which supports the men, the horse, or the automobile, is placed nearer to the knees than to the shoulders. Enormous weights can be supported in this position because most of the weight comes right over the knees, and is supported by the upright bones in the calves of the legs. Since the arms are straight, the bones of the forearm and upper arm are in one line, and each arm, in this position, is capable of sustaining a thousand pounds. I saw Sandow do this stunt with three horses on the plank and I have seen other men support automobiles. What the record is I don't know; but I have seen a 125-lb. woman support 2000 lbs. in this "human-bridge" position, and I believe that any amateur barbell user, after a few months' experience, could support over 3000 lbs.

The foregoing stunts are more in the class of supporting feats than lifts. Another supporting feat is the one shown in Fig 19, but instead of using a bar-bell the professional will hold on his feet a long plank and on this plank will be seated a dozen men. Supporting a great weight is easy in this position, after the legs are straightened; but as I said in Chapter IV, the strength of a man's thighs is so prodigious that a well-trained lifter can hold 1500 lbs. on the soles of his feet, as in Fig. 19, and then raise it an inch or two by straightening the legs. Saxon used to do this with close to 3000 lbs.; that is, he would first lie flat on his back and raise his legs in the air. His younger brothers would then put the plank on his feet. Fourteen of the circus attendants would stand with their backs to the plank, and the two younger Saxon;

would pick up these men in pairs and seat them on the plank. After they were all in position, Saxon would bend his legs and lower the weight a couple of inches, and then again straighten his legs. Two of the Saxons used to lie flat on their backs and hold a bridge or the soles of their feet and a very heavy automobile would be run over the bridge.

The strength of the bones of the hips is something phenomenal A well-trained bar-bell user can lift anywhere from 1000 to 1500 lbs. by the "hip" lift, which has already been described in Chapter V. After the weight has been raised by straightening the legs, you can then straighten up the body without much difficulty If you stand erect, with the legs straight and the feet a few inches from each other and firmly braced, it takes a tremendous weight to make you bend your legs again.

The first exhibition work of which I ever heard was performed by a German nearly two hundred years ago. In one of his stunts he would stand on a high platform. Around his hips was a strong belt, and from this belt a chain went through a hole in the upper platform; and its bottom end was hooked to a large cannon which weighed over a ton. This cannon rested on a wooden platform which, in turn, rested on a pair of rollers, The athlete stood with his legs straight at the start. The stage attendants would knock the rollers from under the lower platform and the athlete would stand there with the cannon hanging from the chain which was attached to the belt around his hips. Note that the man did not lift the weight, he merely supported it. As he was a very large and powerful individual, he undoubtedly could have lifted 2200 or 2400 lbs. in a "hip" lift; so it was perfectly reasonable to believe that he could have supported nearly twice that much after the legs were straightened. This man invented a lot of other "strength" stunts in the nature of supporting feats, and those stunts are performed on the stage up to this very day.

A professional "Strong Man" should not be blamed for giving a performance of this character. His business is to perform a sensational act; and it stands to reason that the average audience will be much more impressed if he uses weights that can be counted by the ton, rather than weights that can be counted by the hundredweight.

I do not want to give you the impression that any man can get up and do the sensational supporting feats that we see on the stage, because it takes a great deal of bodily strength to give such a performance. The thing you should learn is that many of the stunts which appear to be performed by the strength of the arms are really performed by the strength of the whole body. The average man can't lift 500 lbs. from the ground, and if he tried to walk with that weight on his shoulders, his legs would buckle at the knees and he would crash down in a heap; but a trained man like Matysek or Sandow can stride along easily while supporting 500 or 600 lbs. on the upraised arm. In men like these two, the back and the legs are so strong that it is a simple matter to carry several hundred pounds on the upraised arm.

If your back and legs are strong, you can stand erect and hold a great deal of weight on your shoulders. Fig. 103 shows an amateur walking with about 900 lbs. supported on his shoulders. If this young man stood erect with his legs straight, as the man is doing in Fig. 104, he could support 1500 or 1800 lbs.; but here he is walking with close to 1000 lbs. As has already been told, Barre walked several yards with a 1450-lb. bar-bell on one shoulder, and it is possible that he could have walked with 2000 lbs. across both shoulders.

You can't get the strength to perform supporting feats just by pushing dumbbells or bar-bells to arms' length above the head. To do supporting feats, you need enormous back strength and leg strength; and to develop that kind of strength, you have to practice the leg and back exercises described in Chapters II and IV. After a few weeks' practice of those exercises, you would be able to give quite an impressive show, if you were asked to appear at some amateur entertainment or at a Y. M. C. A. carnival. Back and leg strength will help you more in the ordinary duties of life than will arm strength alone; and that is why I am so insistent on the necessity of creating bodily strength by developing the back and legs.

After you have created strength, you should know how to use it to the best advantage. The combination of your strength and skill will enable you to handle four times as much weight as will the average husky day laborer. For instance, if you saw a bunch of workmen amusing themselves at noon hour by an impromptu lifting contest, you would find that they were using the ordinary "deadweight" style; that is, they would put the weight to be lifted in front of them and stoop over, as in Fig. 14. Then they would stand erect and hold the weight as in Fig. 15. . This is what we call the "dead-weight" lift. Most of the workmen would be unable to stand up in this way with 350 lbs., but if you had developed your back and legs by performing the exercises in Chapters II and IV, you would probably be able to stand up with 450 or 500 lbs. But if you wished to show them what really could be lifted, you could employ the "hand-and-thigh" method, illustrated in Fig 16, or the "Jefferson" lift in Fig. 18, and amaze those workmen by lifting 1000 or 1200 lbs. a couple of inches from the ground.

Never let your enthusiasm for "putting up" bar-bells make you neglect your practice of the leg and back exercises; because leg and back exercises make bodily strength, and it is bodily strength which appeals to the average man. In a football game, when a burly player gains ten yards while carrying four or five of the opposite players on his shoulders and back, he is doing a great feat of bodily strength, and just as admirable a feat of strength as if he were walking with a 1000- or 2000-lb. weight across his shoulders. The great thing is that if you practice back- and leg-lifting, you can develop just the kind of strength which would enable you to make 20-yard gain while dragging or carrying half a dozen of the other team; the kind of strength that would enable you to lift one end of an automobile, and to do other stunts of that kind.

The professional "Strong Man" is an adept at this kind of work. He is the very last word in combined strength and skill. Most professionals are very different in private life than when on the stage. I know some of them who would prefer to give a straight lifting act, but if they did that it would mean that they could get no engagements. Therefore they have to do sensational stunts, and the theatrical manager has a great habit of exaggerating the amount of weight which the athlete uses in the act. If a "Strong Man" tells the manager that he is going to support or lift 2000 lbs. in a certain way, the manager will go immediately to the printing office and get out posters saying that the athlete is going to lift 5000 or 6000 lbs. in that manner.

The manager of a vaudeville theater has the fixed delusion that no one will come to see a "Strong" act, unless the athlete is billed as "The Strongest Man in the World." Hence, every new "Strong Man" at his first appearance is billed in that way. In the last twenty years I have seen at least fifty different professionals, each and every one of whom claimed to be "the strongest man on earth." At the present time, there are seven professionals making that claim.

CHAPTER XXI

WHO IS THE STRONGEST MAN IN THE WORLD?

It is impossible for any one to pick out an individual and say, "This man is stronger than any other human being in the world." The world is a very large place, and there are hundreds of "Strong Men"; some of them professionals, and many more of them amateurs. It is impossible to ever determine who is the strongest man; because, in the first place, it would be impossible to bring all the "Strong Men" of the world together; and in the second place, it would be very difficult to arrange a program of strength tests which would be fair to all the competitors, skilled and unskilled.

When a man is extraordinarily strong, it frequently happens that he is lured into the professional ranks. Consequently, the best known "Strong Men" are professionals. Several years ago I wrote an article for the Physical Culture Magazine, in which I stated that the three strongest men of recent times were Louis Cyr, of Canada; Apollon, of France, and Youssoff, the gigantic Turkish wrestler. I should have qualified that statement by saying that these were the three strongest men who appeared publicly. There are men in Canada today who swear that the amateur, Horace Barre, was just as strong as his professional friend, Louis Cyr. Mr. Jowett says that the amateur, La Vallee, is stronger than either Cyr or Barre were. Apollon was a contemporary of Cyr's. The two never met in a contest. Prof. Des Bonnet, the French authority, claims that Cyr and Apollon were stronger than any other men of their time; but the Professor is a Frenchman, and so was Apollon, while Cyr was of French descent. Youssoff, as far as I can learn, was as strong as either of these two Frenchmen, and possibly stronger. The Germans and Austrians have several claimants for the title, and there is today in Vienna an Austrian named Carl Swaboda, who can beat any one in the world in two-arm bar-bell lifting, and lifting with two arms requires more bodily strength than lifting with one arm at a time. Swaboda is the only man in athletic history who has raised aloft more than 400 lbs. in the two-arm "jerk." His record far excels that of Cyr and Apollon. In Finland they breed a race of giants, and in that country there are undoubtedly men who, for brute strength, can compare to the best of any other nation. Eastern Canada is full of "Strong Men," and for that matter, so is this country. I have seen amateurs who could equal the strength feats of any professional on record, if they cared to devote as much time to training as the professional does. A man does not become strong because he is a professional lifter. It is just the other way about. He becomes a professional because he is strong. And it should be remembered that for every "Strong Man" who exhibits professionally, there are a dozen others in the amateur ranks. I am personally acquainted with three amateurs of prodigious strength, who are as magnificently developed as any of the perfect men you have ever seen on the stage. Not one of these men will allow me to publish his picture, or even mention his name. One of these men has a 48-inch chest, a 16-inch forearm and a 19-inch calf measurement. I once saw him pick up an 80-lb. steel bar, muscle it out, and then twist the bar from side to side; and I have never seen a professional who could equal that stunt. Another of these men is so strong that he can break any of the "deadweight" lifting records. The third man is only of moderate size and weighs but 165 lbs.; but I believe he can walk with more weight on his shoulders than any other man I have ever seen.

There has never been a man so strong that he could far outdo the feats of other "Strong Men." What one man can do, another man in the same class can go very close to equaling. If you get the five best sprinters in the same 100-yard dash, the best man will finish only a foot ahead of the second man; which means that he is only a fraction of one per cent faster. If the best high- jumper can clear the bar at 6 feet 6 inches, the second and third best can do 6 feet 5 inches. The same rule applies to "Strong Men." As a class, these men are two or three times as strong as the ordinary man; but no one "Strong Man" is very much better than other leading "Strong Men." Some of them excel at one lift, some excel at others. Arthur Saxon could push aloft with one arm a bell 20 lbs. heavier than any other man has lifted in the same manner, but there were a number of men who could beat him at a two-arm lift. Steinborn is possibly the best man in the world at what we call the "quick lifts"; but there are men who can beat him at "slow-pressing," and other men who could undoubtedly beat him at "dead-weight" lifting; and so on down the list.

You can't even decide the question by examining the records. To publish a complete list of lifting records would take several dozen pages of this book, because they keep the records for men of all weights and for all styles of lifting. Many of the world's records are held by amateurs. Joe Nordquest, when still an amateur, broke records made by the professionals, Hackenschmidt and Lurich. The same thing applies to weight throwing. Most of the records for throwing the hammer or throwing the 56-lb. weight are held by amateurs. There is no reason in the world why an amateur should not be just as strong as a professional. You would be surprised if you knew of the thousands of men who by practicing lifting just for the sport of it have become magnificently built.

A strength contest is something like these newspaper beauty contests. Every once in a while you see in the papers the picture of some young woman who has taken first place in a beauty contest, and who is announced as "the most beautiful woman in America." And when you see that picture, you say to yourself, "I know half a dozen girls better-looking than she is." The truth of the matter is, that she happened to be the best-looking girl in that particular contest, or at least the Judges thought so. You know perfectly well that for every pretty girl who goes in such a contest, there are fifty more girls equally pretty who never even thought of entering the contest; and you can rest assured that for every man who is announced as the "strongest man in the world," there are several dozen others who are just about as strong as he is. If you were willing to train, you have just as good a chance as the next fellow to become one of the strongest men in the world of your weight; and if you are of average size, that means that you can become almost as strong as anybody, because I have proved in a previous chapter that men who weigh less than 150 lbs. have come very close to equaling the best records of "natural giants" who weigh 300 lbs. Any man who is willing to devote six months or a year to practicing a progressive schedule of developing exercises can certainly double, and possibly triple, his own bodily strength, and that means that in that length of time he will become two or three times as strong as the average man.

PLATE 71

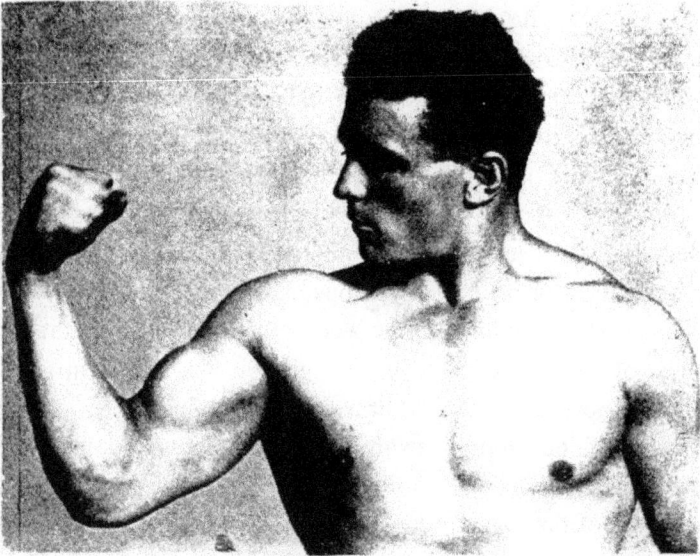

Fig. 142

Plate 71, Figure 142. An attractive pose by Henry Steinborn, one of the greatest lifters in history. Although Steinborn has used bar-bells for years, his muscles, though wonderfully developed, are as long, and as smooth as those of a boxer. His arm, which measures over 17 inches, seems small in this picture, and if you read the chapter on "Muscle Control," you will realize that he could have made his biceps more prominent by raising his arm as Snyder did in Figure 91. But even though his arm is not flexed, the immense width of his shoulders, and the size of his upper-body muscles prove that he is a Hercules

PLATE 72

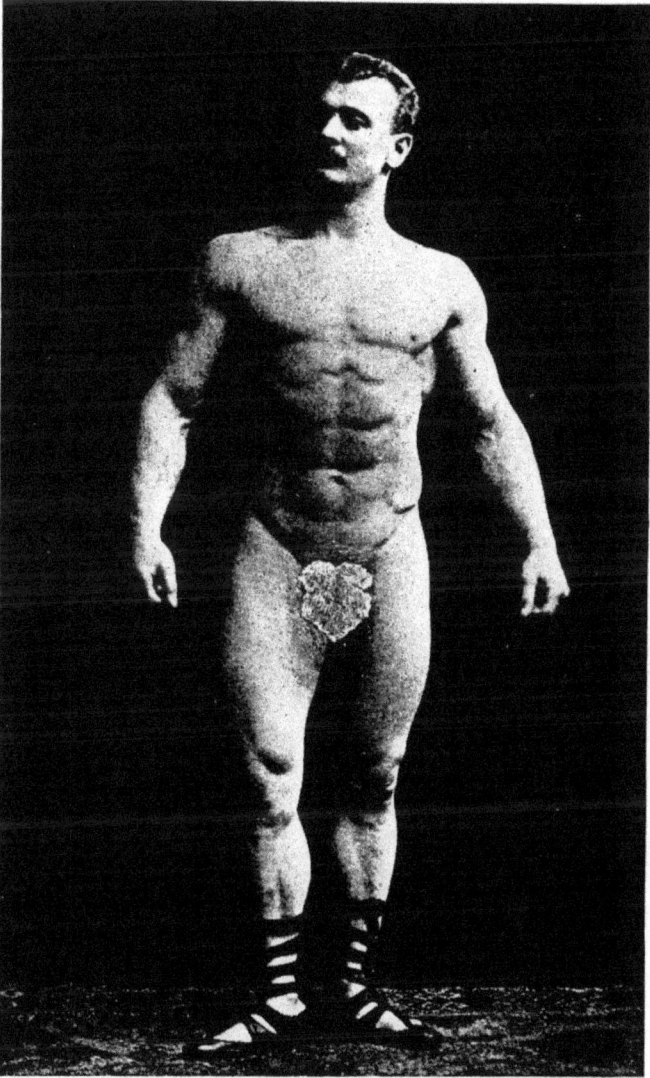

Fig. 143

Plate 72, Figure 143. Sandow standing at ease. It is interesting to compare this picture with some of the others, in which he is deliberately flexing his muscles.

PLATE 73

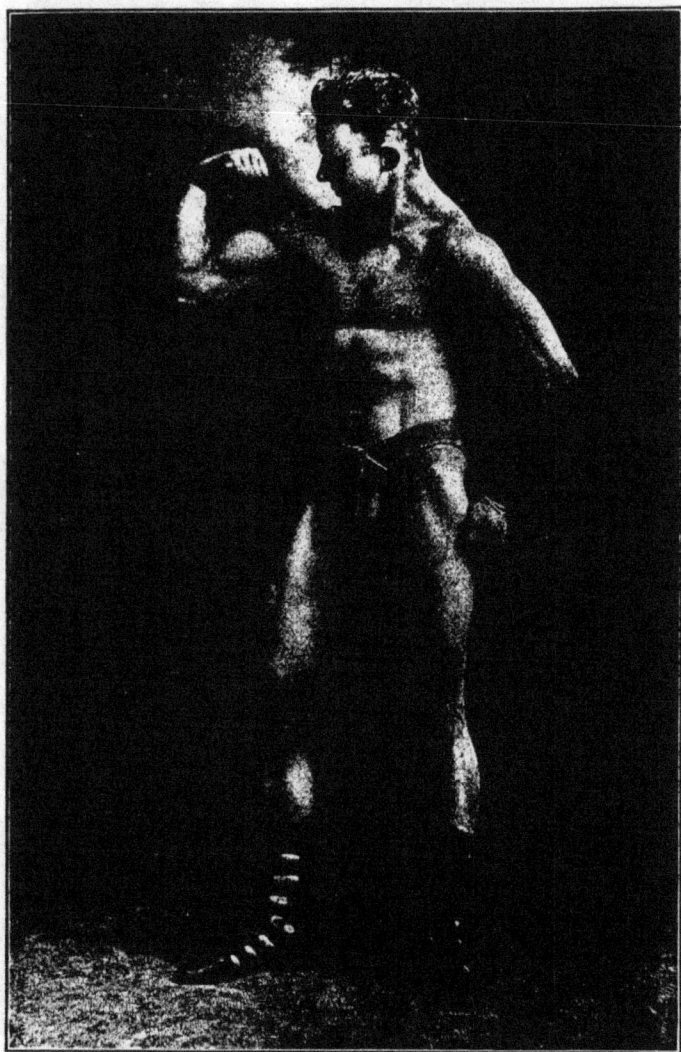

Fig. 144

Plate 73, Figure 144. Owen Carr with muscles flexed. His arm,
chest, neck, and legs show up wonderfully, but the whole effect is
not as pleasing as in Figure 136

PLATE 74

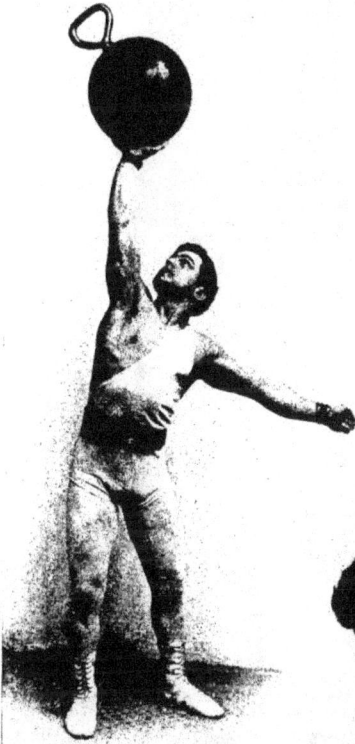

Fig. 145

Plate 74, Figure 145 (above). Ali Kotier, a Syrian athlete, who has made his home in this country. Although he weighs only 140 lbs., he can lift nearly 300 lbs. over-head in the "Two-Arm Jerk." His bodily strength is enormous

Fig. 146

In Figure 146 (below) he is holding a kettle-bell in a way that shows off his beautiful shoulder and biceps muscles. From this position he threw the bell straight up in the air, and caught it on the palm of the right hand, as in Figure 145 (above)

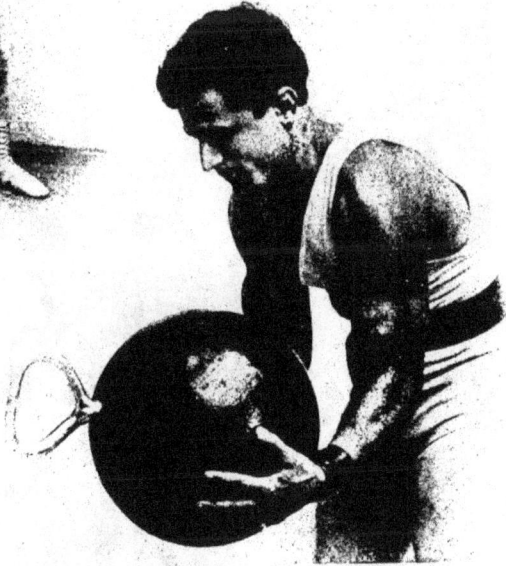

PLATE 75

Fig. 147

Plate 75, Figure 147 (a b o v e). Joe Nordquest at the time he made the world's record for an amateur, by lifting 277 lbs. aloft with the left arm, using the "B e n t Press" method. (I n practice he has more than once pressed 300 lbs.)

Fig. 148

Figure 148 (below), will give you an idea of his prodigious chest a n d arm development. His forearm flexed measures 16 inches, and his upper arm flexed nearly 18 inches

PLATE 76

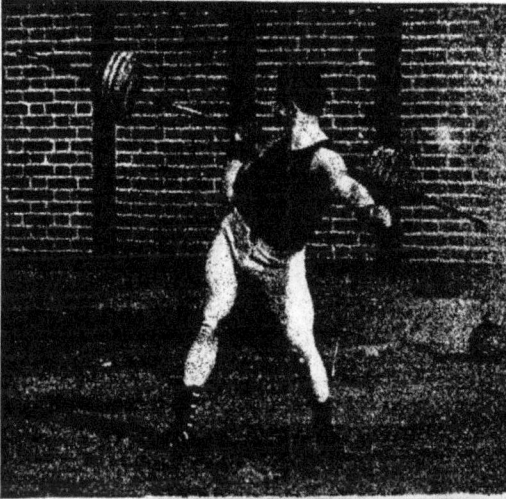

Fig. 149

Plate 76, Figur
149 (above)
Matysek startin
a right arn
"Bent Press
with a 235-lb
bar-bell. Thi
pose is an inter
mediate stag
between Figure
111 and 112
The picture wa
snapped just a
he started t
bend. Figur
150 (below)
Matysek doing a
"Shoulder
stand" with a
220-lb. bar-bell

Fig. 150

First he lay
flat on his
back, lifted the
bell with the
hands, and
placed it on
the soles of
his feet. After
he straight-
ened the legs,
he raised the
hips from the
ground, and
did the "Shoul-
der stand" as
shown. Every
muscle in his
legs is flexed
in the act of
supporting the
weight

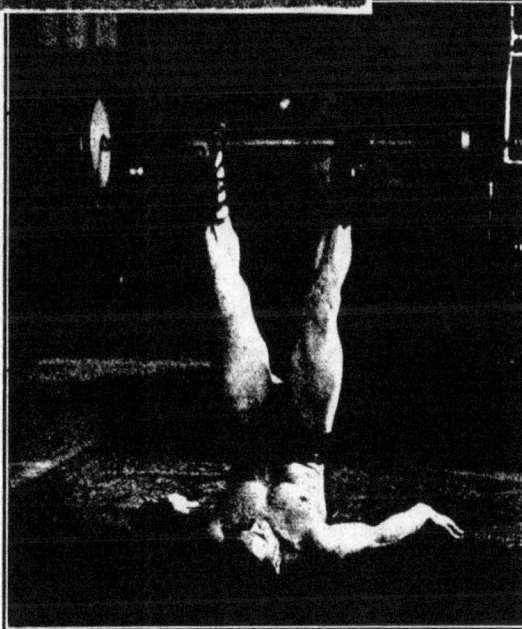

PLATE 77

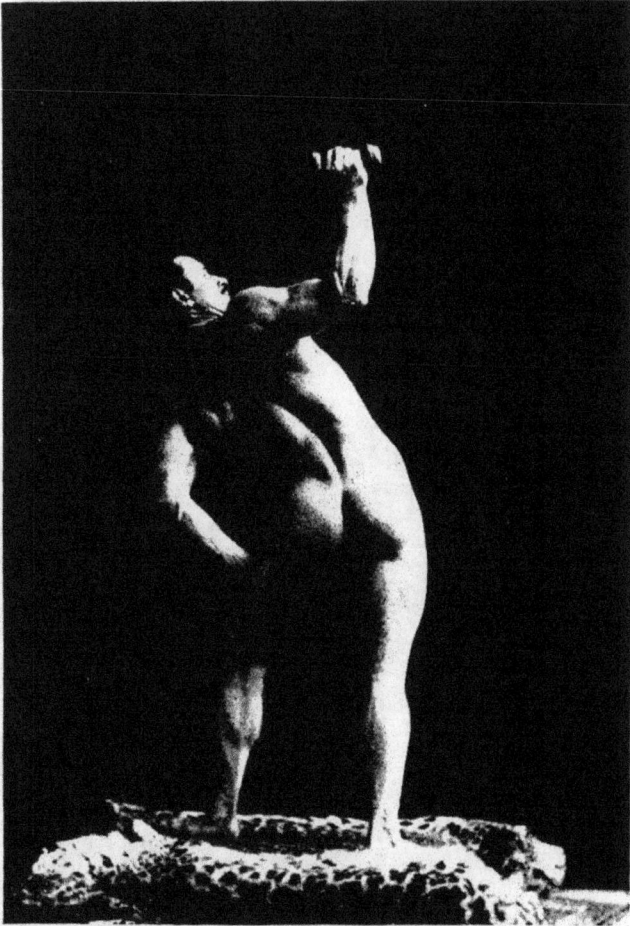

Fig. 151

Plate 77, Figure 151. A photo by Sarony, showing Sandow
demonstrating a one-arm "Press". A beautiful pose which
proves that the more correctly a man lifts, the more graceful
will be his position

PLATE 78

Fig. 152

Plate 78, Figure 152
(above). Klein do-
ing a one - arm
"P r e s s" with a
h e a v y dumbbell.
(Compare this pic-
ture with the pose
of Sandow, Figure
151.)

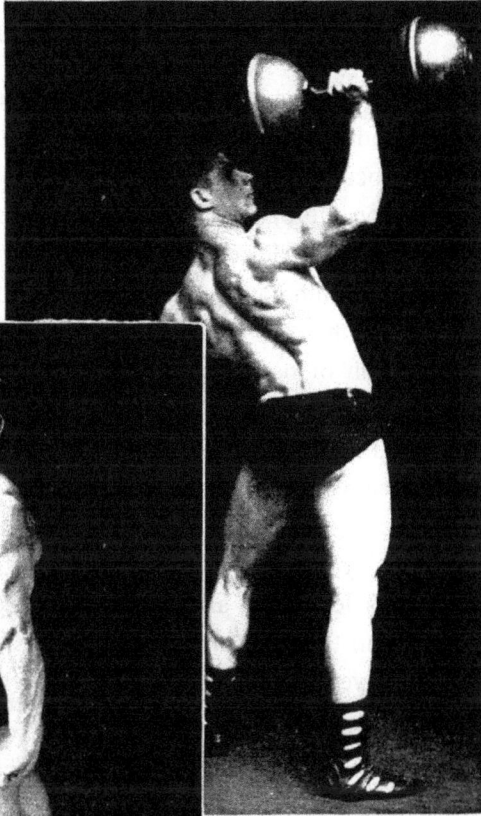

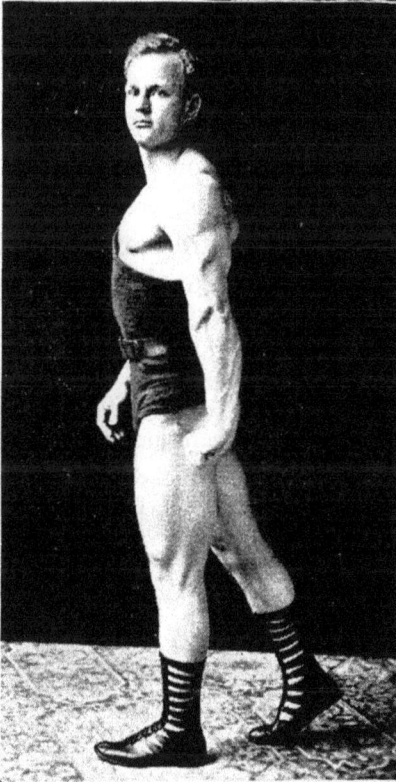

Fig. 153

Figure 153 (below).
Edward Gokenbach, a
young amateur bar-bell
lifter, who has a phy-
sique of the Viking
type

229

CHAPTER XXII

MORE ABOUT LIFTING

Besides the various lifts described in the previous chapters, there are many other varieties of lifts which are practiced more or less. In some localities, there is a vogue for lifting bar-bells while lying fiat on the back. The lifter lies with the bell on the floor beyond his head. He reaches backward, grasps the handle of the bar-bell with both hands, lifts it across the face, and then raises it to arms' length, as in Fig. 105. Such a lift is more a test of arm strength than of bodily strength, but because the shoulders are supported by the floor, it is possible to push more weight to arms' length than when the athlete is standing erect on his feet. Also, when you're lying on your back, you push the bell in a different direction than you do when standing erect. When on the back, you practically push the bell in front of you, and the triceps muscles of the arms can exert more strength in pushing forward than they can in pushing upward. The record for a two-arm "pull-over" and "push" was held for many years by George Hackenschmidt, with 361 lbs. In making this record, he used a bar-bell with spherical ends, and each sphere measured 19 inches in diameter. The spheres were so big that Hackenschmidt did not have to do much lifting to get the bell across his face to above his chest, because the handle was so high from the ground that all he had to do was to lean his face sideways. After he got the bell to the chest, he shoved it aloft easily by pure arm strength. On November 8, 1916, I saw this record broken by Joe Nordquest. In order to put him on equal terms with Hackenschmidt, I made some iron plates 19 inches in diameter. The bell was first loaded to 300 lbs., and gradually increased until it weighed 363 lbs. At that weight Joe pushed the bell aloft without any great exertion.

Arthur Saxon discovered that it was possible to push much harder with the arms if, instead of lying flat on the back, the body was arched in a shoulder bridge. His record was 386 lbs., and Joe Nordquest broke it at my factory on February 17, 1917, by lifting 388 lbs. in the same style, which is shown in Fig. 168.

There is still another style of lifting, known as the "body-toss," which is also performed while the athlete is lying on the floor. After he has pulled the bell across the face, he rolls it down the body until the handle rests right across his stomach. Then he bends his legs, places the soles of his feet on the floor, and raises his body in what we call the "shoulder bridge," that is, supported just by the shoulders and feet. To make the lift, he lowers the hips, and then quickly raises them and elevates the bell by a toss of the body and by a quick push of the arms. Lurich holds this record with about 420 lbs.

The third lift in this class is known as the "wrestler's bridge" lift. Before the lifter pulls the bell from floor to chest, he arches his body into a "wrestler's bridge," bearing all his weight on the soles of his feet and the crown of his head. Then he pulls the bell over the face, and slowly presses it to arms' length, as in Fig. 106. Hackenschmidt holds this record with 320 lbs. This lift requires great strength in the back and the neck, as well as tremendous lifting and pushing power in the arm muscles. This lift can be converted into an attractive supporting feat. The hard work is pushing the bell to arms' length. After the arms are straightened, a great weight can be supported, either by the arms or on the body. Fig. 106 shows Owen Carr making a "wrestler's bridge" lift with 296 lbs., while Fig. 107 shows him supporting a total weight of 560 lbs. in the same position.

When I gave a list of developing exercises in the first part of the book, I did not include any for the neck. You can get all the special neck development you want by practicing lifting in the "wrestler's bridge" position, and it is not necessary for you to tyro break any records. You can start with as low as 30 or 40 lbs. and by the time you have become able to pull a 100-lb. bell to the chest and then push it aloft six or eight times in succession, your neck will become as round and as well-shaped as you could possibly desire.

I have found that the neck increases in size and strength when using bar-bells, even if you do not take any special exercise for the neck itself. If a man starts out with a 36-inch chest and a 17-inch shoulder width, his neck will probably measure 14¼ inches. If, by practicing developing exercises, he increases the size of his chest to 42 inches, and his shoulder width to 20 inches, his neck will increase to 15½ inches, or possibly to 15¾ inches, at the same time, even if he has not done one exercise for the neck muscles. The size and shape of your neck is a barometer of your vitality; the face is the barometer of your condition. If your cheeks sag, it is a sign of poor condition, because that facial condition means that your body muscles are flabby. If your face is so thin that your cheeks are hollow, and if there are circles under your eyes, it means either that you are undernourished or overtrained. You can always tell a man's condition by looking at the contours of his face and the brightness of his eyes. In the same way you can tell the mount of vitality a man possesses by looking at the shape and size of his neck. If his neck is round as a column and shows no particular muscle, except under exertion, then he possesses a great amount of vitality. Any gain or loss in vitality is immediately revealed by an improvement, or the reverse, in the appearance of his neck.

CHAPTER XXIII

SOME OUT-WORN SUPERSTITIONS

I can state positively that the easiest and quickest way to get a magnificent build, and the super-strength that goes with it, is to practice a progressive schedule of developing exercises with an adjustable bar-bell; but if your friends learn that you contemplate training with a bar-bell they will endeavor to dissuade you. You will be told that using bar-bells will make you slow and "muscle- bound," will make you die young, that it will strain your heart, etc.

Years ago, when I first got interested in bar-bell work, I was told just these things, and I admit that I used to worry about them and wonder whether or not they were true. When your friends tell you these things, it is likely that they will sincerely believe all the things they say; and so, their objections are worthy of serious consideration. You cannot dispose of an opponent's arguments just by saying that what he says is not true, and that what you say is true. You should have some facts on which to base your arguments, and happily, I have those facts. I admit that some of the popular ideas about bar-bell exercise are supported by the experience of the lifters and "Strong Men" who were produced in this country from fifty to seventy-five years ago. In those days, there was no such thing as an adjustable bar-bell, that is, one which could be easily and quickly changed in weight. All they had were short-handled, solid dumbbells. The big gymnasium would probably have a pair of 25-pounders, a pair of 50-pounders, one 75-pounder, one 100-pounder, and possibly a still bigger dumbbell, weighing 150 pounds. With these bells, the athletes could do only a limited number of exercises, and those exercises developed only the muscles of the arms and shoulders.

Practically all they did was to slowly "curl" a dumbbell from the hip to the shoulder, in order to develop the biceps muscles, and then "push" the dumbbell overhead, in order to develop the triceps at shoulder muscles. With such dumbbells as they owned, that was about all they could do; or at least all that they knew how to do. seems they knew nothing whatever about any of the "quick lifts," any of the exercises which develop the chest itself, or which strengthen the back, or which develop the legs. Their idea seems to be that with a pair of heavy dumbbells, you did exactly the san exercises which you would do with a pair of 5-lb. dumbbell (As a matter of fact, there are still many people who cling to the idea, thinking that if you use heavy bar-bells, you take one in each hand and go through a drill consisting of many arm movement the way you do when you're using a pair of light dumbbells.)

If a man did take a 50-lb bell or a 75-lb. dumbbell and practice half an hour or an hour, and just did "curling" a bell and pushing it aloft, I can quite see that his arms and shoulders would be developed out of all proportion to the rest of the body, and if he made his practice too strenuous the arm and shoulder muscles could become stiffened, and, consequently, slow in action. I understand that such cases happened, although they were before my time and I have never seen a man so stiffened.

I can also understand that if a man had only solid dumbbells 1 work with, and, consequently, was unable to adjust the weight or the bells to suit his strength, he might quite possibly overexert himself, and overexertion frequently results in heart strain.

These old-timers who trained in the manner above describe were tremendously handicapped. They reaped but few of the benefits which can be gotten from the intelligent use of the present-day adjustable bar-bell. Such strength as they obtained was entirely in their arms and shoulders, and, consequently, many of them were top-heavy in build. Notwithstanding the fact that the specialized on arm exercises, they never were able to realize thrown possibilities in the way of bodily strength, nor to do as much with their arms as they should have done. Their "curling" and

234

"pressing" records seem like kindergarten stunts compared with the records of the modern lifters.

Nevertheless, a few very strong men were developed in the middle of the last century in this country, and the surprising thing is, that most of those "Strong Men" in their own cases contradicted all the accepted ideas; that is, instead of being slow and "muscle- bound," dying young, and having weak hearts, they were unusually speedy, lived to a great age, and had no heart trouble whatever.

The first great American "Strong Man" was a certain Dr. Winship, who lived in New England. The first great American advocate of bar-bell lifting was Thos. Wentworth Higginson. Mr. Higginson was a very prominent literary man of his time, and instead of writing for an athletic magazine as you might expect, he happened to contribute to the Atlantic Monthly. He used to take a great pleasure in recounting the sensational strength feats of Dr. Winship, and he advocated the use of bar-bells and weights, not for the means of record making, but as what he called "health lifts." Mr. Higginson was far ahead of his time. Apparently, he was the first man to realize the possibility of creating great bodily strength by lifting really heavy weights by the strength of the back and legs.

I don't know what became of Winship, nor how old he was when he died; but I do know that he did all kinds of lifting, and that he was prodigiously strong. Following Dr. Winship came two gentlemen by the names of Curtis and Buermeyer. The first named was known in his later years as "Father Bill Curtis," and for a great many years before his death he was connected with the Amateur Athletic Union, and probably did more than any other individual to popularize track and field sports. In his youth, Curtis was a great user of dumbbells. According to the old record books he took in each hand a 100-lb. dumbbell, "curled" them slowly to the shoulders and "pushed" them slowly aloft. To "push' that much weight is a stunt that any modern amateur can do with ease; but "curling" 100 lbs. in each hand is a great feat of strength Curtis lifted about 3600 pounds in a "back" lift. He was big and tremendously powerful; but his bulk and great development did not prevent him from making an official record of 10 seconds in a hundred-yard dash. When he died, Curtis must have been 55 or 60 years old. He and a friend named Ormsby made an ascent of Mt Washington, were caught in a blizzard and frozen to death. Up to the time of his unfortunate accident, Curtis apparently retained most of the activity and most of the strength he had as a youth.

His friend and contemporary, Mr. Buermeyer, was also a great sprinter and a great lifter. I believe this gentleman died a year or two ago, in Brooklyn, at the age of 83, and it was said that even when he was 80 he would practice regularly with a 100 lb. bar-bell. The use of bar-bells did not seem to affect either the speed, the health, or the heart strength of these two men.

I became actively interested in bar-bell work in 1902. At that time I was instrumental in persuading a lot of young men to take up bar-bell exercises, and I am happy to say that almost all of these men got great results from their exercises; that is, they became very much bigger, stronger, well developed and healthier. I am still in touch with most of those men, who are now at, or past middle age; and I am happy to say that those men have retained their great strength and development, and that they seem to be just as healthy and just as active as they were when they finished their first training with bar-bells.

In 1902 there were several well-known professional and amateur lifters who must have been between 30 and 40 years old at that time. Those men, while they have retired from active competition or exhibition work, are still living, and each one of them is still two or three times as strong as the average. No one of them seems to have suffered any of the ill effects which the use of bar-bells is supposed to produce.

In the Strength magazine for April, 1924, I wrote an article about my friend, Mr. George Zottman, who first appeared as a professional lifter about 1890, who retired a few years later, and who today, at the age of 57, is a physical marvel. His picture is shown in Fig. 109. Another man, a little older than Zottman, is John Y. Smith, of Boston. There are few men in athletic history who have ever done as much lifting as this man. Smith retired from professional work in 1903, when he was 37 years old. One of his friends, hearing that Smith had retired, said to him, "Now that you have stopped lifting big weights you will go to pieces and die soon." "Nonsense!" replied Smith, "I will meet you here when I am 50 years old, and I will put up 200 lbs. with either hand." An argument ensued and a bet was made. In 1911, when 45 years old, Smith emerged from his retirement and gave a wonderful exhibition of lifting. On his fiftieth birthday, in 1916, he happened to remember the bet, and determined to win it. As he had not even touched a bar-bell since 1912 he put in a few days training, and a few days after his fiftieth birthday he went to the gymnasium and put up a 203½-lb. dumbbell first with the right hand and then with the left hand. Early in 1924 I had a letter from one of my Boston correspondents, who said that Smith still occasionally went to the Y.M.C.U. in Boston, and that he had recently seen him making a one-arm "push-up" with a 200-lb. dumbbell. Pretty fair for a man of 58! Smith's picture is shown in Fig. 110. That picture was taken twenty years ago; but his friends say that it would be a good picture of him today, and that although he takes but little exercise he still retains his figure and his immense strength and energy.

When it is said that a man has an "enlarged heart," it does not necessarily imply that his heart has been damaged. In some cases enlarged heart is quite serious, because, as a result of some strain, the wall of the heart has been stretched, and thereby became weaker and thinner; or it may be that the heart has been enlarged in way that affects one of the valves, so that it no longer fits, and thus causes a leakage.

The walls of the heart are of muscular tissue, and if one train correctly, it is possible to thicken and strengthen the heart wall; just as you thicken and strengthen an exterior voluntary muscle If a man builds up his exterior muscles he should build up his heart muscles at the same time. The condition just described is known as true, or concentric, hypertrophy. A heart so developed will be somewhat bigger and stronger than before, and there is not the slightest danger of that heart deteriorating after a man stops training.

Heavy exercise of any kind makes a great demand on the lungs and bar-bell work is no exception. By performing the leg and back exercises described in Chapters II and IV, you can increase your lung power just as easily as by long-distance running. One of the first things that a beginner must learn is to breathe in rhythm with the movements when he is exercising. He should breathe in as the muscles are contracted, and breathe out as they are relaxed or vice versa. If in any exercise the body is bent at the hips, it is wisest to breathe out as the body is bent, and breathe in as it is straightened. For example, when doing a back exercise like the one shown in Figs. 10 and 11, you should breathe out as you bend over, and breathe in as you stand up, because as you bend over the body is compressed in a way that leaves you less lung room. In the same way, when doing the abdominal exercise shown in Fig. 36, you should breathe out as you bend and raise the body and breathe in as you lower the body.

Never attempt to hold the breath while making several successive and vigorous motions, because if you did that the effect on the heart would be just as bad as when swimming under water. When making a very heavy lift it is sometimes necessary to exhale and inhale several times during the course of the lift. Some lifters have the business of breathing down to a science; as, for example, Mr. George Jowett who, when making a one-arm "bent press," breathes in at three separate stages.

There is a theory that one can exert more strength when the lungs are full of air. This is true in regard to some bar-bell lifts, because if the chest is slightly expanded and the air retained in the lungs for these few seconds while the arm is being used, the ribs are held in one position, and so the muscles attached to the ribs have a stationary, instead of a moving, anchorage, and can be flexed with greater force.

There is a popular superstition to the effect that the use of heavy bar-bells is hard on the heart; yet I, who have known (and still know) thousands of lifters, have never known one man who contracted heart trouble from the use of bar-bells or in doing actual lifting.

One of the causes of heart trouble is overstrain, but heart trouble can be caused by under feeding and holding the breath just as easily as by any overexertion. In your experience you have frequently heard references to the so-called "athletic heart," and it is possible that you, like many others, may believe that indulgence in any form of athletics causes a permanent lesion of the heart. From what I can learn swimming produces more cases of heart trouble than any other kind of sport, because in swimming all the muscles are used simultaneously, and the breathing has to be done in a certain way. Nevertheless, a man can swim moderately for years and never injure his heart the slightest. It is when competing in swimming races, and particularly in swimming under water that heart strain takes place. It is the height of folly to make continued vigorous exertions at the same time you are holding the breath, and for that reason I consider swimming under water to be the most dangerous of sports.

In the same way a man may practice running for the exercise he gets out of it, and actually build up his heart and make it stronger. If a man strains his heart through running, it is almost always as a result of taking place in some strenuous race in which he forces himself to continue long after he is exhausted. The hardest of all competitive sports is rowing, especially the four-mile college boat races. No man with a weak heart has any business in a racing shell; although a man with a weak heart would never last long enough to win his place in the boat. Although the exertion is strenuous in the extreme, it does not seem to cause heart trouble. An investigation proved that college rowing men lived longer on the average than the non-athletic members of their classes, and in this investigation they collected statistics on classes that had graduated as long as fifty years ago.

Heavy gymnastic work does not cause heart strain, and neither does bar-bell work.

I understand in the history of lifting there have been two or three men who have broken a blood vessel or sustained heart failure when making some strenuous lift. I say that I understand this to be so, because I have never been able to find the names of those men.

Progressive exercise with an adjustable bar-bell is just about the safest of all ways of making yourself big and strong. This is because every sensible person who uses a bar-bell naturally adjusts it to weights that he can handle with ease and comfort, and he increases the amount of weight he is using only when his increased weight and development shows him that it is safe to do so.

In this respect bar-bell exercise has many advantages over gymnasium work. If you go to a gymnasium and try to develop yourself by practicing vigorous stunts on the swinging rings, horizontal bars, the parallel bars, etc., you have to handle the weight of your body in every stunt. You find that either you can lift or support your weight, or else you cannot, and in the second case it is impossible to make yourself lighter by cutting off an arm or a leg. With a bar-bell you can readily adjust the weight to suit the strength of one muscle, or of any other muscle or set of muscles. With a combination-set you can adjust the kettle-bells to fifteen or twenty pounds for arm exercises, and a minute later you can be practicing heavy back-and-leg exercises with the bar-bell form adjusted to three or four hundred pounds.

Suppose you and a number of other men had agreed to get together and build a tennis court. Your job might be to trundle a wheelbarrow and transport dirt from one part of the court to another. If you were told three or four days in advance that such was to be your job, you would not consider it necessary to do a whole lot of light exercise as a preparation; but when the day came you would report with your sleeves rolled up ready for work. If, after wheeling a few loads, you found that the other fellows were overloading the wheelbarrow, you would say, "Look here! You're making this thing too heavy. Put less dirt in this time." Your protective instinct would immediately assert itself. You would know that if the wheelbarrow was overloaded to such an extent that it made you struggle along, you would overexert yourself, and you might strain your back. Therefore, you would do the sensible thing and move the dirt by making more trips with less weight each trip. In using a bar-bell you do exactly the same thing. If you attempt an exercise or lift and the weight seems to be too heavy, you immediately reduce the weight by removing some of the iron plates until you get a weight which you can handle with a fair amount of ease, and with benefit to yourself. In the old days when they had nothing except solid dumbbells, a lifter did not have this advantage; and if a man of that period hurt himself, it was probably because he tried to push up a 150-lb. dumbbell when he was strong enough to push up only no lbs. Having nothing between 100 and 150 lbs. he had no choice.

I have heard of some men straining their backs or their shoulders by lifting heavy bar-bells or dumbbells, but invariably these were men who were using a bar-bell for the first time. It has always seemed very strange to me that the average man is very reluctant to admit that he is less strong than any of his friends. He will willingly admit that some big stranger may be stronger, but he will not yield the palm to any of his friends, especially if they are about his own size. If a crowd of young fellows happen to come across a 100-lb. dumbbell, and one of their number "puts it up," every other man in the crowd will have a try at it; and in that case it can easily happen that one or two of them can strain their shoulders or back. It is just as foolish for an untrained man of average size to attempt to push up a 100-lb. dumbbell with one hand, as it would be for a non-swimmer to jump off a ferryboat in the middle of a deep river and try to swim ashore; or as foolish as it would be for you to try to ride a hundred miles the first time you got on a bicycle. When you learn swimming you do not start in forty feet of water, but at a four-foot depth; when you start to ride a bicycle you first have to learn to stay on, and then for a few days you ride only short distances. When you start to use a bar-bell you should apply the same principle. You begin with your bar-bell adjusted to light weights and by gradually increasing the weight, build yourself up. After a few weeks or months of such training, you will become so strong that you can handle large weights with ease, and with perfect safety.

There are people who claim that if a man uses bar-bells for a certain time and then stops his training, he will go to pieces physically. I have never known this to happen. I correspond with a large number of lifters, and hardly a day passes that I do not get a letter from some man who says, "Although I had not used my bar-bell for fifteen years, I picked it up the other day and found that I could lift just about as much as when I was in regular training." And most of them say that they still keep the development they got from their bar-bell exercises. The most interesting case of this kind is that of George Zottman (previously referred to), who retired from the stage nearly thirty years ago, who still keeps his 46-inch chest, his 34-inch waist, his 18-inch arm, who has gained only five pounds in weight, and who is today, at the age of fifty-seven, one of the strongest men in the country. He used his bar-bells continuously up to the time that he was 30 years old, but since then he has not touched a bar- bell oftener than twice a year.

Why should a man "go to seed" physically because he stops his exercise? As far as I can find out, the idea seems to be that during his training his organs have been overworked in the effort to support his muscular development, and that when he stops his hard muscular work his organs continue to work at the same pace as before; and that in some mysterious way this causes the man to suddenly decline in health. For the life of me I cannot see why this should be so. I know men who did the hardest kind of labor as young men, who changed the character of their work when they became about thirty, and who today as elderly men are just as vigorous as ever. For example, one of my friends is the superintendent of a rolling mill. In his youth he was a roller, and made steel rails. With a pair of tongs he would pick up one end of a very heavy iron rail and put it between the rollers. He worked on an eight-hour shift, and in the course of a day's work he would handle more tons of iron than a bar-bell user would handle in a month. He spent his young manhood at this job. At twenty- eight he became foreman, and at thirty-five was superintendent. Today he is over sixty, and he is as vigorous a specimen as you would want to meet. This man when a roller had a killing job. He stopped it abruptly, but that stoppage did not seem to make him go to pieces or to make him any less healthy. I have known bar-bell lifters to have just the same experience. They would first spend a year in getting a wonderful muscular development; then for a couple of years they would be very much interested in actual lifting and would spend considerable time at it. Then they might move to some other town or take a job which made it impossible for them to continue their lifting. In the course of my business I see such men every day, and so far as I can see they enjoy just as rugged health as they did when they were training, and there is no sign of any deterioration in their lungs, heart or kidneys. If I had space and it was worthwhile, I could fill the remainder of this book in giving you the names and describing the development and accomplishments of such men. I do not have to theorize on this subject because there is such conclusive proof constantly before me. If you will give the matter consideration, I think you will admit there is no reason why a bar-bell user should go to pieces any more than a rowing man should go to pieces when he abandons his daily practice on the river. As a matter of fact, strength once made stays with you practically the rest of your life; and the stronger you have made yourself, the longer that life is apt to be.

In conclusion, I admit that competitive lifting by absolutely untrained men can easily be dangerous, but then—there is very little competitive lifting, and there is absolutely no need for a man to take part in such contests unless he wishes to. As I have said several times before in this very book, it is much better to use bar-bells as a means of building up your body than to use them for the purpose of making lifting records.

Boxing enthusiasts are apt to tell you that the use of heavy bar-bells will make you slow and "muscle-bound." There seems to be some mystery connected with that last phrase. Personally, I have never been able to find out what is just meant by the term "muscle-bound." If you will ask five of your friends what they mean by those words, the chances are that each one of the five will tell you something entirely different. The general idea seems to be that when a man is muscle-bound his muscles are so big, and so stiff in action that he is unable to move about with any degree of freedom. I suppose there is such a condition. If a coal-heaver stands in a bent-over position and shovels coal for two hours without stopping, you will notice that when he finally drops his shovel he will have considerable trouble in standing erect. His back muscles have become so tired through the continued labor that the act of standing erect has to be performed very slowly, and seems to be accompanied with considerable pain. You might call that being "muscle-bound"; and I believe it is true that men who do that kind of work gradually get in such a condition that they are permanently stooped. I believe that this condition comes from maintaining the body so long in one position, because the oarsman who uses his back just as vigorously does not seem to suffer the same effects. But then, the oarsman straightens his back at the finish of each stroke, whereas the coal-heaver rarely stands erect as he wields his shovel. As I said previously, I believe that if a man took a dumbbell weighing say seventy-five or a hundred pounds, and spent quite a time each day in just pushing it aloft, he could eventually stiffen the shoulder muscles just in the way that the coal-heaver's back muscles became stiffened. It happens that I have never seen such a case, although I have heard such cases did occur in the early days of lifting.

When Sandow first came to this country he caused a sensation by his muscular development. In his stage act he lifted enormous weights, and some critics, who admitted that his development was undoubtedly due to bar-bell exercises, circulated the story that he was so "muscle-bound" that he could not raise his hands far enough to adjust the collar button at the back of his neck. I suppose there were people who believed that story. The fact was that Sandow's muscles when at rest were as pliable and elastic as the muscles of a light-weight boxer; and Sandow was almost as supple as a contortionist, as well as being as quick with his hands as a professional juggler. I saw him turn a back somersault with a fifty-pound dumbbell in each hand; and he had his ankles tied together, and was blindfolded. A back somersault under any conditions requires great suppleness and agility, but under Sandow's conditions it required what you might call super-agility. You can see how he looked when relaxed in Figure 143.

The adept at modern lifting has to possess unusual speed for movement, for without such speed he cannot make respectable records. I have never seen another two hundred and fifteen-pound man who could equal the lifter Steinborn for sheer speed of movement. Refer back to the section of the lifts known as the "snatch" and the "jerk," and you will see that at a certain point in those lifts it is necessary to completely change the body position, and that change has to be effected in a very small fraction of a second. Steinborn's speed was simply dazzling. Consider the time that he made the two-arm jerk with 347 pounds. The first shove of his arms and legs carried the bell about as high as the top of his head. Before it had the chance to drop a quarter of an inch, Steinborn had squatted to his heels and had his arms perfectly straight under the bell. He changed from a standing to a squatting position with such speed that it seemed magical. He had to be quick. There he was for an instant with 347 pounds at the level of his crown. Either he had to get under the bell or else it would crash to the floor; and you can take it from me that it does not take long for a 347 pound weight to start to drop.

Another happening on the same evening gave another demonstration of Steinborn's speed. Like many foreign-trained lifters, he was in the habit of letting the bell fall to the floor if he

246

saw that he was not going to successfully "fix" it. He attempted the one-arm snatch with 218 pounds. If he had accomplished it, it would have been the biggest "snatch" ever made in America. The first heave sent the bell all the way from the floor to arms' length, but the tremendous effort threw him slightly off his balance. Realizing that he could not hold the bell without danger of over-balancing, he let go of the handle bar and hurled himself to one side. The bell came down with a crash, but by the time it hit the floor, Steinborn was sitting against a wall ten feet away.

(This might make you believe that when you use a bar-bell it is necessary to continually drop it. If you are practicing a "snatch" or the one-arm bent-press, you can learn to lift a greater weight if you are doing your lifting in some place where you can drop the bell without damaging anything. When you are doing developing exercises and moderate lifting, it is never necessary to drop the bell. Thousands of men today are using bar-bells in their own bedrooms. You can use a bar-bell in any space where you have room enough to use a pair of five-pound dumbbells, and when using your bells you need not be afraid that anybody in the next room or in the room below you will hear you exercise or notice any vibration. It is just as easy and just as safe to exercise with a bar-bell in your own room as it would be for you to learn to do the one-step in the same room.)

PLATE 79

Fig. 154

Plate 79, Figure 154 (above). Edward Goodman, an attorney of Los Angeles, creating a record by lifting 107½ lbs. in the "Abdominal raise." (Same as the exercise shown in Figure 36.)

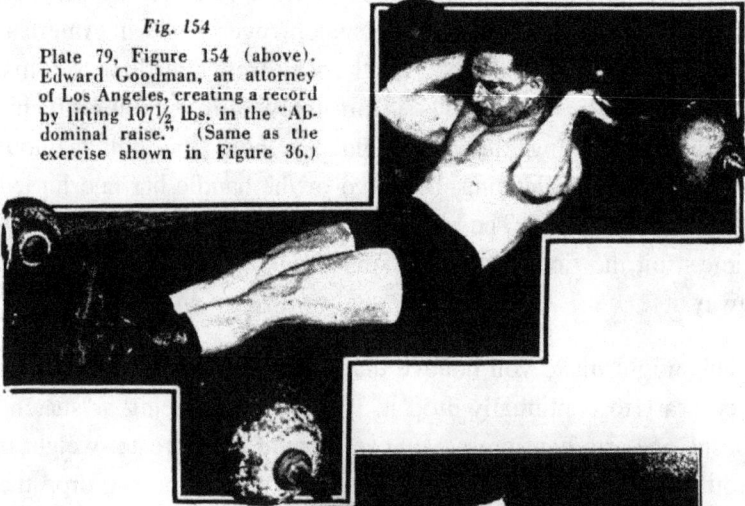

Fig. 155

Figure 155 (below). A picture of Goodman showing his extraordinary arm and shoulder development. This man has light bones, as is shown by the small size of his hips, and the trimness of his joints. His chest measurement is very much larger than his waist measurement

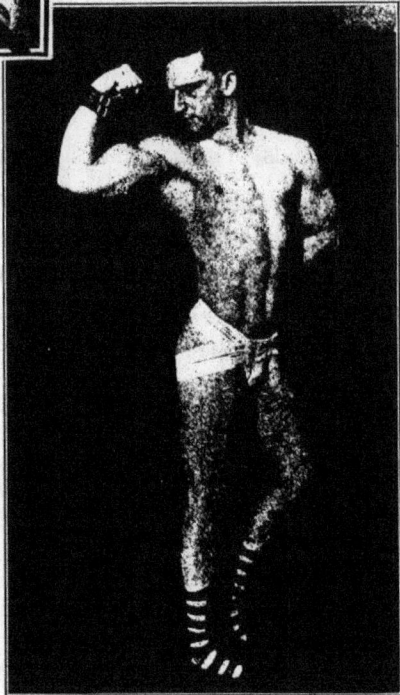

248

PLATE 80

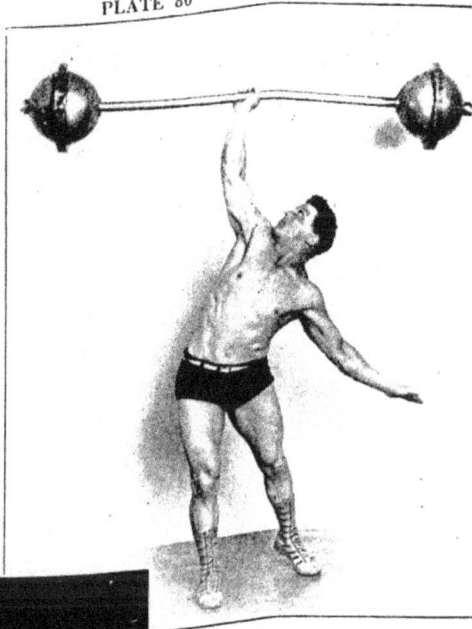

Fig. 156

Plate 80, Figure 156 (above). Henry Steinborn, at the finish of a "One-Arm-Snatch." The bell used weighed 173 lbs., and had a handle 1½ inches thick. On this occasion he snatched the weight six times in succession.

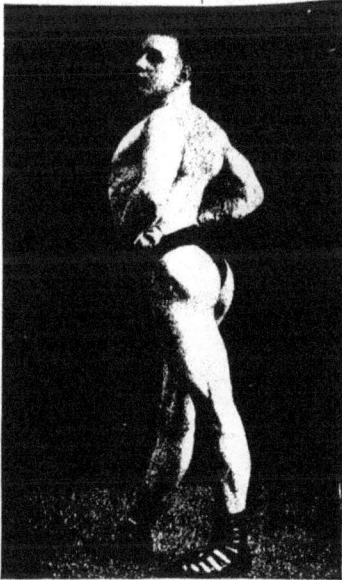

Fig. 157

Figure 157 (below). George Lurich, the famous wrestler and weight-lifter, who holds the world's record in the lift known as the "One-Arm-Jerk." This is the man who walked while carrying five men overhead at the full stretch of his right arm.

PLATE 81

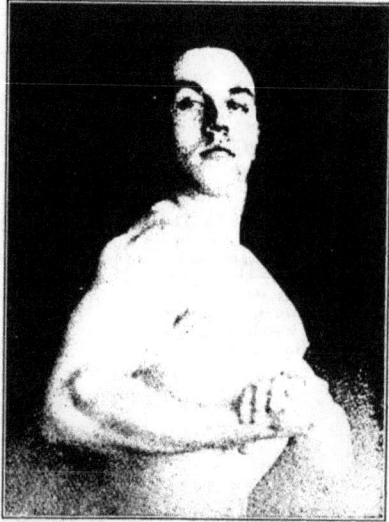

Fig. 158

Plate 81. Melvin Tampke, an amateur from San Antonio, Texas. Figure 158 (above), was taken at the age of twenty, after he had been training about a year. By a combination of developing exercises and actual lifting, he obtained a 45-inch normal chest, a 16½-inch upper arm, and a 24-inch thigh. His best record in the one-arm "Press" was 235 lbs.

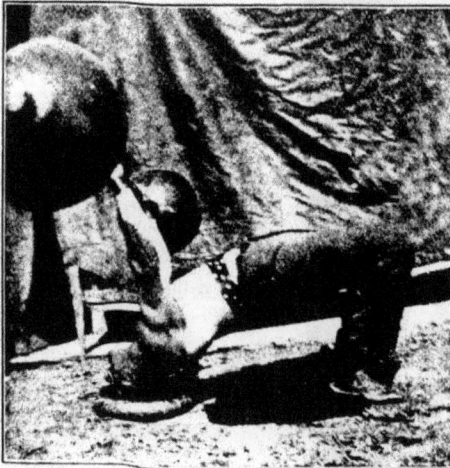

Fig. 159

Figure 159 (below), shows him making a two-arm "Press" in the "Wrestler's bridge" position. The bar-bell shown in the picture is the one used in making his one-arm "Bent Press" lift.

250

PLATE 82

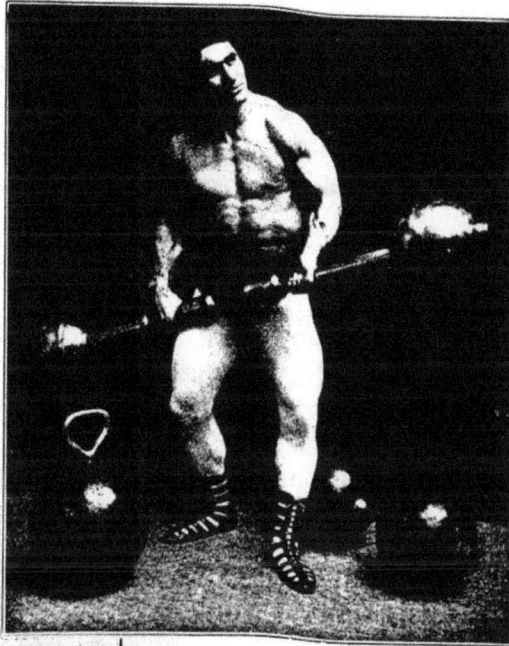

Fig. 160

Plate 82, Figure 160 (above). Tony Massimo poses with a lot of exhibition bells. This picture was taken when he visited my factory in 1916. Besides being a fine lifter, this man was one of the very best hand-balancers on the professional stage

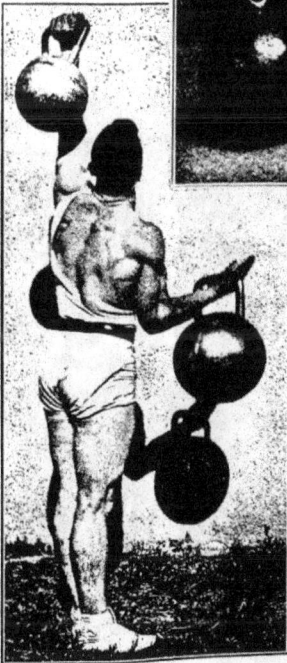

Fig. 161

Figure 161 (below). Albert Tauscher in an unusual pose with two kettle-bells. The interesting part of this picture is the clean-cut appearance of the deltoid muscle at the point of the right shoulder. This muscle, which raises the arm, is called into vigorous action when you push a weight aloft, or when you hold a heavy weight in the hand. In Figure 160 you can see how Massimo's left deltoid is made to stand out by the downward pull of the bar-bell which he is holding in his hands

251

PLATE 83

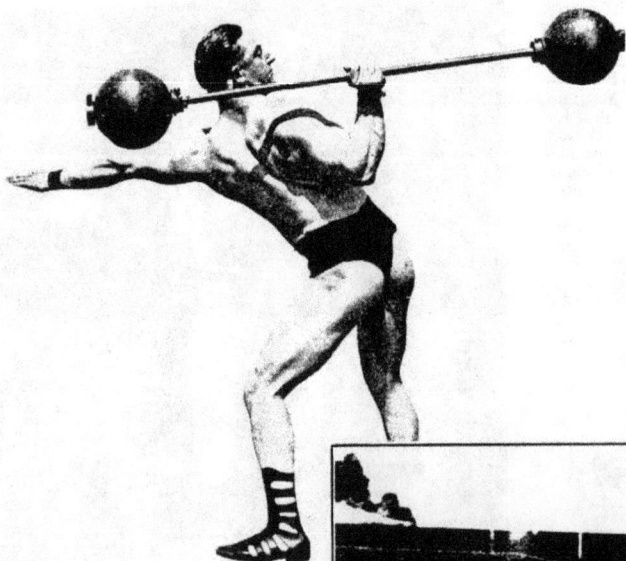

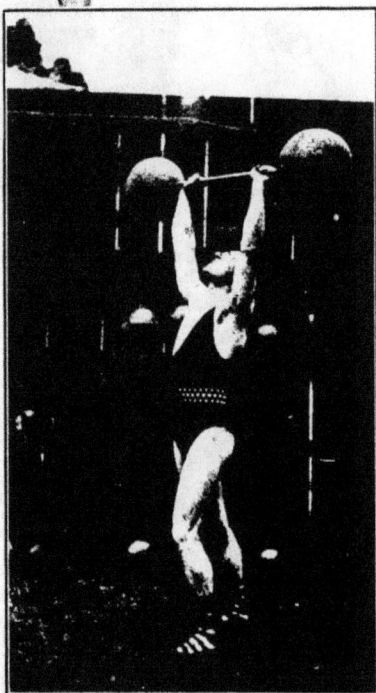

Fig. 162

Plate 83, Figure 162 (above). Edward Goodman starting a one-arm "Bent Press"

Fig. 163

Figure 163 (below). L. M. Littrell, a San Francisco amateur, who stands five feet ten inches in height, has a 43-inch normal chest, a 15½-inch biceps, and has raised 226 lbs. in a one-arm "Bent Press"

PLATE 84

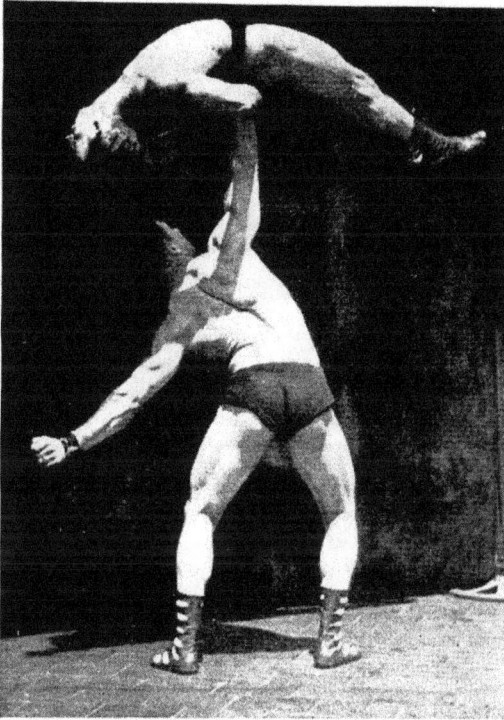

Fig. 164

Plate 84, Figure 1
(above). A sna
shot of Sigmu
Klein, showing hi
making a one-ar
lift with a 135-l
man. Notice h
closely his bodi
position in this p:
ture compares
his position in Fi
ure 152

Fig. 165

Figure 165 (below).
A snapshot of Klein
displaying his arm and
upper-back muscles.

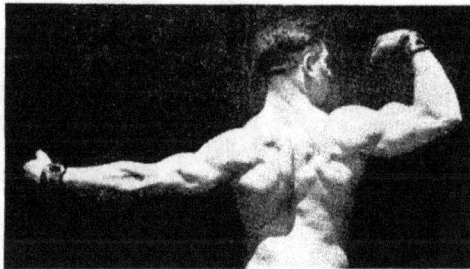

PLATE 85

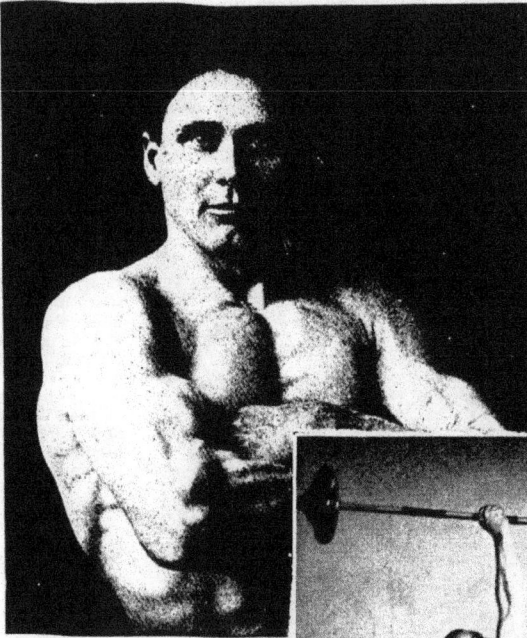

Fig. 166

Plate 85, Figure 166 (above). John Y. Smith, of Boston, a picture taken twenty years ago. Although fifty-eight years old at the present time, he can still make a one-arm "Press" with 200 lbs.

Fig. 167

Figure 167 (below). Roy L. Smith, the New York amateur, at the finish of a one-arm "Press." This man took up lifting at the age of thirty. When he began his practice he could not put up 60 lbs. with one hand. As before stated, his record in this lift is now 245 lbs.

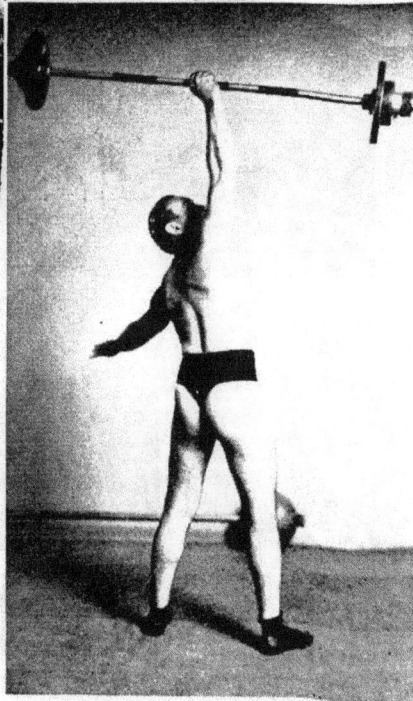

PLATE 86

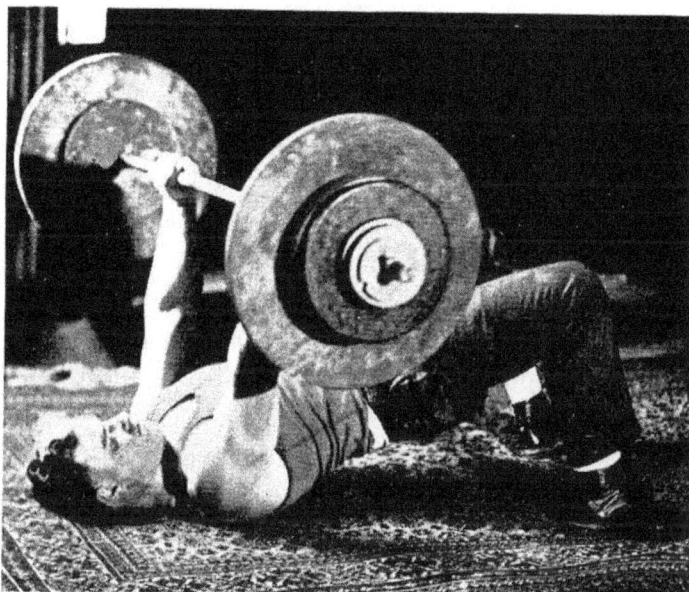

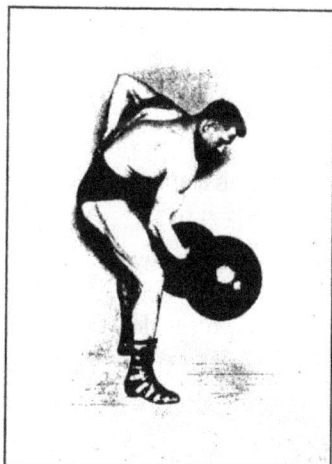

Fig. 168

Plate 86, Figure 168 (above),
shows Joe Nordquest making
a world's record by pressing
388 lbs. to arms' length while
in the "shoulder-bridge" position. This lift broke Arthur
Saxon's record of 386 lbs.

Fig. 169

Figure 169 (below). Anton
Matysek making a "One-Arm
Curl" with a big "exhibition"
dumbbell

CHAPTER XXIV

THE SECRET OF THE BENT-PRESS

The "bent-press" is a combination of bodily strength and acquired skill. It is not a lift which a man will do instinctively— he has to be taught. It is possible to lift so much more weight by this method than by any other, so the lift is well worth learning. When you reflect that Arthur Saxon, whose best record in the military press was about 126 lbs., could raise 336 lbs. when he used the bent- press method, and that Sandow, who could military press only 121 lbs., could bent-press 271 lbs., you get an idea of the possibilities of the method. A star at the bent-press will raise two and a half times as much by that method as he can if he stands erect in the military style and pushes the weight up just by the strength of his arm and shoulder. If you can make a military press with a 50-lb weight you can, by learning the method, make a bent-press with anywhere from 125 to 150 lbs. The Englishman, Pullum, when he weighed less than 126 lbs., raised 86 lbs. with the right arm in the military style, and 216 lbs. in the bent-press style. Another lightweight Englishman, who weighed 120 lbs., pressed something like 221 lbs. A number of comparatively small men have succeeded in lifting, by this method, a bar-bell which weighed 100 lbs, more than their own body weight. Since Saxon weighed about 210 lbs. when he bent-pressed 370 lbs., he did 160 lbs. more than his own weight.

Any real expert at the bent-press can press aloft more weight with one arm than he can with two arms; and there are some men who can raise almost as much in the one-arm bent-press as in a two-arm jerk. If you can make a one-arm military press with 50 lbs., the chances are that you can make a two-arm press (not military) with no or 115 lbs.; and, as I have said before, if you master the method you can make a one-arm bent-press with 125 lbs. or more. The odd thing is that it actually takes less exertion to bent-press 125 lbs. with one arm than to make a two-arm press with 115 lbs.

Whoever it was who said that the bent-press was a matter scientific body leverage, described the lift exactly. In making a bent-press the lifter supplements the strength of his arm and shoulder by the strength of his back, his sides, and his thighs, as well as utilizing the strength of his bones. When a novice first attempts the bent-press he will almost invariably try to shove the bar-bell upwards by a fierce pressure of the lifting arm. The proper way to start the bent-press is to get into the position shown in Fig. 111. The lifter stands with the heels 18 or 20 inches apart, and the toes turned out, so that the feet are at right angles to each other. After he has lifted the bell to the height of his shoulders he thrusts his right hip out to the side, bends his body slightly to the left, and rests his right elbow on the top of the right hip bone. If you take this picture, Fig. 111, and hold a ruler over it, you will see that there is a straight line running downwards from the right hand to the right heel. There is no exertion necessary to hold the bell, because the weight is supported on the vertical bones of the right forearm, and that is in turn supported by the bones of the hip and the bones of the right leg. Some of you may have difficulty in getting your elbow on the hip, because you will try to lean directly sideways, instead of leaning slightly to the left and slightly to the front. (The bar-bell should always be turned as shown in the picture; that is, with the handle almost parallel with the shoulders.) By putting the elbow on the hip, the right arm is pressed against the right side of the body.

Now, the lifter leans to the left and forwards; that is, his body rotates slightly on its own axis as he bends. He places the inside of his left forearm right above the left knee as he bends over, and he has to be particularly careful to keep the right arm from sliding off the right side. (In Fig. 112 you cannot see the inside edge of the right arm, but I can assure you that it is still supported by the right side.) As the lifter bends over he keeps his right forearm straight up and down, since the right upper arm is still resting on the right side, it means that the arm is "opened."

In Fig. 113, which is next in order, the lifter has bent a little further over, and now you can see his right upper arm resting on his right side. Since the forearm has been kept perpendicular to the floor, it is now at right angles to the upper arm. The left forearm has been slid along the left thigh into the position shown, By pressing the left forearm firmly against the left thigh the lifter gets an artificial support. Without that support there would be a great strain on the muscles of the right side of the waist, and on the small of the back.

In the fourth position, Fig. 114, the lifter has leaned so far that the right arm has almost straightened itself. He has shifted his left forearm again so that the left wrist is against the thigh, The left arm is completely doubled, but it still acts as a support. Now, for the first time, the lifter commences to push hard with the right hand, so as to straighten the right arm. At this point of the lift his body is firmly braced by the support afforded by the left leg and the doubled up left arm.

Fig. 115 is the last in the set, and shows that the lifter has finally succeeded in straightening the arm. The problem now is to stand erect and complete the lift. The customary way to accomplish this is to bend the right leg at the knee, which thereby lowers the right hip and brings the lifter into a sort of a crouch beneath the bell. Assisting himself by pressing hard with his left hand, the lifter stands erect, and the lift is completed.

If the bent-press is properly performed there is no great strain felt in any of the muscles, except at the stages between Fig. 114 and 115.

Now, to support my statement that the bell is not actually lifted until after the arm is straightened, I invite a closer inspection of the pictures showing the start of the lift and the end of the lift. Measure Fig. 111 (the start) and make a note of how many inches there is between the right hand and the right heel. Take Fig. 114, when the lifter has his arm almost straight, and measure the distance between the right hand and the left heel. Unless I am greatly mistaken you will find the two measurements identical. This proves that the bell has not been lifted. It is held at one height and the lifter gets his arm straight by bending the body over.

This is as concise a description of the bent-press as I can give. There are many fine points connected with the lift, and to describe them all would take many pages. I can briefly mention, as one of the important details, the swinging of the bar-bell. Between Fig. 111 and Fig. 115 the bell has swung through almost a half circle; that is, the end which was originally in front of lifter in Fig. 111, is now behind him in the last picture. As he stands up the bell will swing back to its original position.

No two men will perform the bent-press in identically the same way. There is always a slight variation in the placing of the feet, in the way the right arm is supported on the right side, in the way the body is bent, etc. Nevertheless, all lifters have to conform to the general laws of position. The Germans call this lift the "screw press," because the left shoulder travels downward in a descending spiral motion, like the thread of a screw, or like a handrail of a spiral staircase. The body is never bent directly to the side, but sideways and forwards. If you will make the experiment of standing with the feet properly placed, and without any bell in the right hand, and then lean over and place the left shoulder right above the left knee, you will see for yourself the way the body has to rotate as it is bent forward.

Some lifters handicap themselves by not using the left arm properly. They start out by placing it just as this lifter does, but they keep on sliding it further and further across the left thigh until the left arm-pit rests on the left knee. In such a case, the left arm is either waving in the air between the legs, or else the left hand has to be placed on the right knee. This leaves the lifter in an awkward position, and makes it more difficult for him to use his left hand as an assistance in raising his body to the vertical position after the right arm has been straightened. All the foregoing seem highly complicated, and I can assure you that it is complicated. Some of you will never be able to master this lift; while others will "get the hang" of it after a couple of days practice, and will soon be able to lift weights that they cannot press aloft with both arms.

Some of the European lifters will not attempt a bent-press. Neither Charles Herold nor Henry Steinborn considered it as a real lift; yet Arthur Saxon, who was developed in the same lifting-club that Herold came from, practiced the bent-press more than any other lift, and made his reputation by it. It certainly is a spectacular feat of strength, and it is sometimes used by professionals to discourage the competition of ambitious amateurs. A good professional makes nothing of a right arm bent press with 225 lbs. For such a lift he uses a bar-bell with a rather thick handle. If any man from the audience questions the professional's strength, he is invited to take the bar-bell in both hands, and press it aloft. There are comparatively few amateurs who can make a two-arm press with 225 lbs., (that is, the kind of amateurs who make themselves obnoxious) and since it is hard to lift a thick-handled 225 lb. bar-bell to the shoulder, the amateur rarely gets even that far. After it has been demonstrated to the satisfaction of the audience that the amateur cannot raise the bell aloft by the strength of both arms, the professional then

makes a right arm bent-press, showing that he can raise the weight by the strength of one arm.

In this connection, I might say that a first-class amateur lifter very rarely interrupts a professional "Strong Man" who happens to be giving a theatrical performance. The amateur fully understands that the professional is paid to entertain the audience, and that it is necessary to perform lifts which are sensational in character. When an amateur lifter goes to such a performance, it is with the object of learning what he can, by watching the professional perform; and since most of these professionals are highly skilled, in addition to being very strong, there is a lot that can be learned in that way. I have known professionals to give sensational exhibitions every afternoon and evening during a week's engagement, and to spend their morning hours at some local gymnasium or lifting club. When in the "gym," they take part in all sorts of friendly contests, and if some members of the club are skilled amateur lifters, the professional will conduct himself just as one of the group, and together with the other lifters will practice all the recognized standard lifts.

When I found that I needed this set of five pictures, I enlisted the services of a Mr. William Langhorne. He kindly volunteered to pose, in spite of the fact that he had not had a bar-bell in his hand since 1907. He weighs but a little over 140 lbs. He is now forty-five years old, and has not gained a pound in weight since he stopped training seventeen years ago. He is a master of the bent-press, and his best lift in that style is 214 lbs. His best record at the two-arm press is 165 lbs., and in the two-arm jerk about 215 lbs. Mr. Langhorne is not entirely satisfied with the pictures, and claimed that the positions were not exactly perfect, because the bell was not heavy enough to force his body and arm into the correct positions. The bell used in the picture weighed only about 85 lbs., and Langhorne said that this was too light a weight to be properly pressed, and that the pictures would have been

more accurate if the bell had weighed over 125 lbs. When doing the posing, all he seemed to do was to shift his body from one position to another, and the bar-bell apparently went to arms' length of its own accord. The more correctly you do the lift, the easier it becomes. Mr. Langhorne is a great hand-balancer. He lived in England twenty years ago, and one winter he took second place in the "open" lifting-championship, (being defeated by a man who weighed 220 lbs.), and in the same season he won the gymnastic championship; while the following summer he took a dozen first prizes in bicycle racing, and several prizes for sprinting. Today he can do a one-hand stand with the utmost ease. He says that the bent-press is largely a matter of balance, and that any expert hand-balancer, who can do a one-hand stand, should have no trouble in mastering the principles of the bent-press.

I am afraid that after you read all the foregoing, you may conclude that the bent-press is simply a trick, and requires no strength whatever. It does require strength in a high degree, and the more bodily strength you possess, the more apt you are to succeed at the lift. Lifters are apt to speak of a 200 lb. bent- press as just an average performance; but you should not forget that before a 200 lb. weight can be pressed aloft, it first has to be lifted as high as the right shoulder, and held there. Very few of the outsiders who read this book are able to lift 200 lbs. more than a few inches off the ground; let alone raising it as high as the shoulder, and then holding it there in one hand. In order to make a big bent-press, you have to be about five times as strong as the average man in the back, and in the waist.

I am printing a few pictures showing other lifters doing the bent-press. There is one of Matysek, Figure 116, showing that an early stage in his career, he made the bent-press improperly, neglecting to use the left arm as he should. When the picture was taken, he was just failing to lift 215 lbs. I had him coached by an expert, who taught him the correct style, and shortly thereafter

PLATE 88

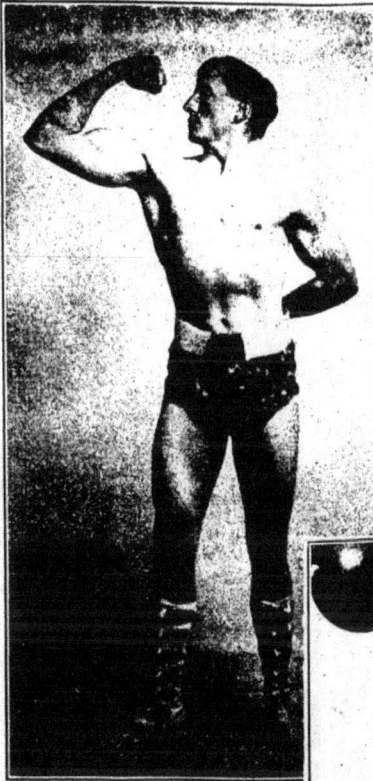

Fig. 171

Plate 88, Figure 171 (above
The Texas amateur, Frank I
Smith, another tall man of tl
slender type, who developed
finely proportioned body l
using bar-bells. Athough h
wrist measures only 7 inche
he managed to develop a 1
inch forearm, and a 15½-in
upper arm, and a normal che
measurement of 42 inches.

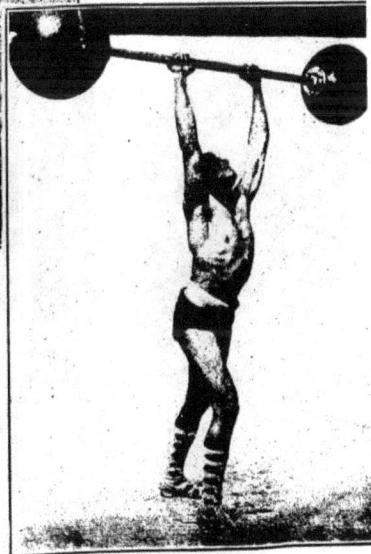

Fig. 172

Figure 172 (below), shows Mr.
Smith finishing a "Two-Arm
Jerk" with a heavy bar-bell

265

PLATE 89

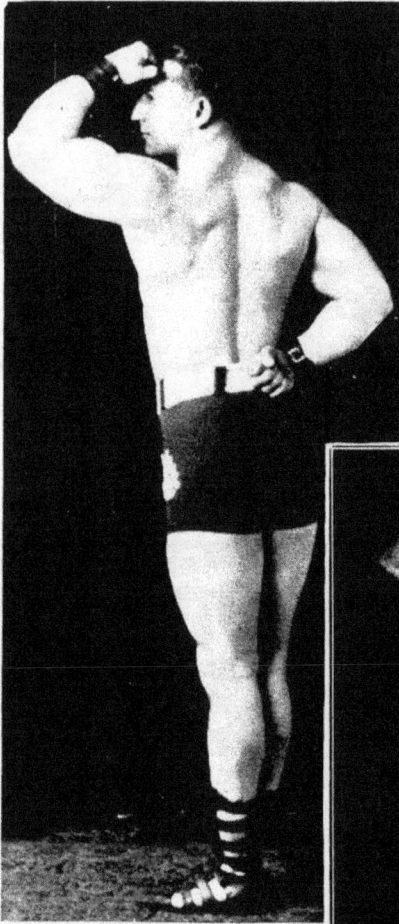

Fig. 173

Plate 89, Figure 173
(above). A recent pic-
ture of E d w a r d W.
Goodman. This gentle-
man is one of the best-
known amateur lifters
in the whole world. In
one afternoon he broke
seven of the British
amateur lifting records

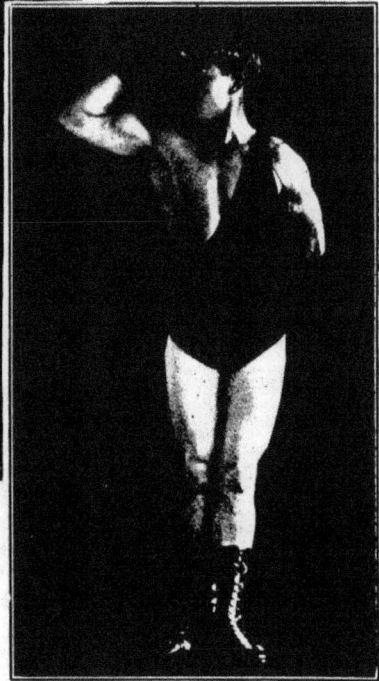

Fig. 174
Figure 174 (b e l o w).
F. R. Rohde

PLATE 90

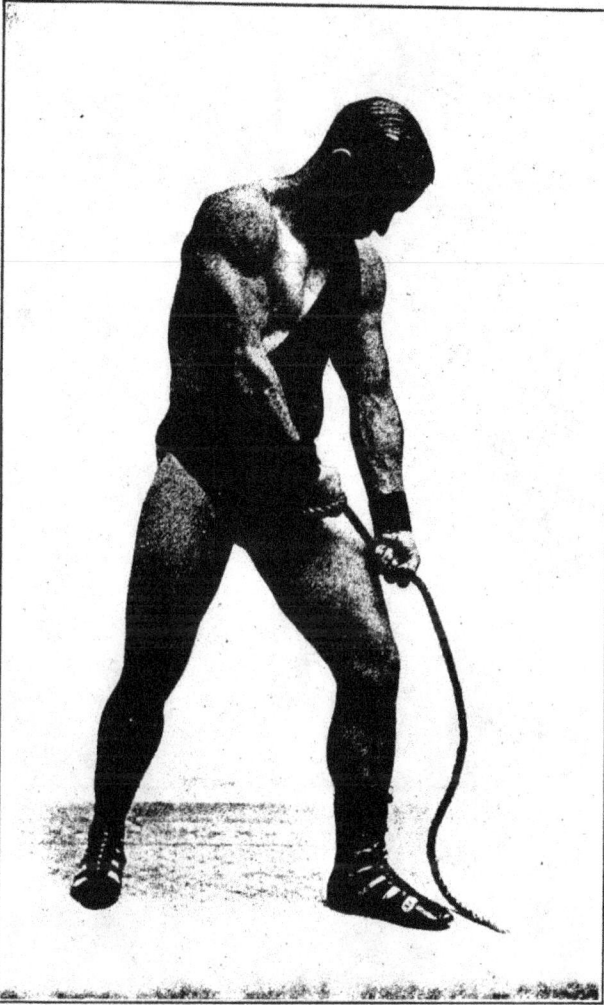

Fig. 175

Plate 90, Figure 175. Charles Durner in a rope breaking pose, which displays the great size of his upper arm and shoulder.

PLATE 91

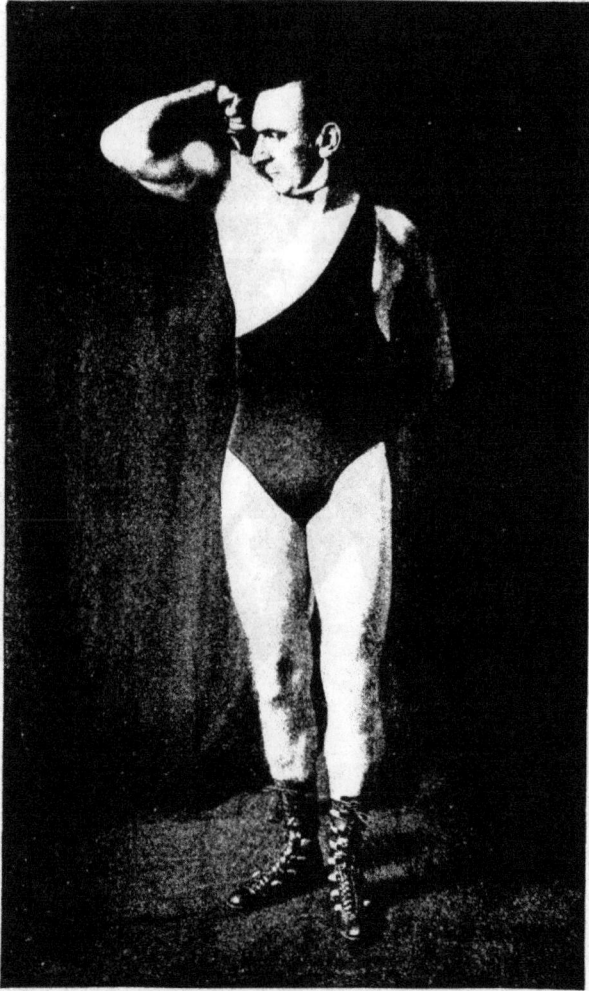

Fig. 176

Plate 91, Figure 176. Roy L. Smith, who, by using bar-balls, increased his chest measurement from 36 to 44 inches, and his upper arm from 12½ to 15¾ inches, and his bodily weight from 145 to 183 lbs. A striking example of what can be done by a man when he starts to train after he is thirty years old.

PLATE 92

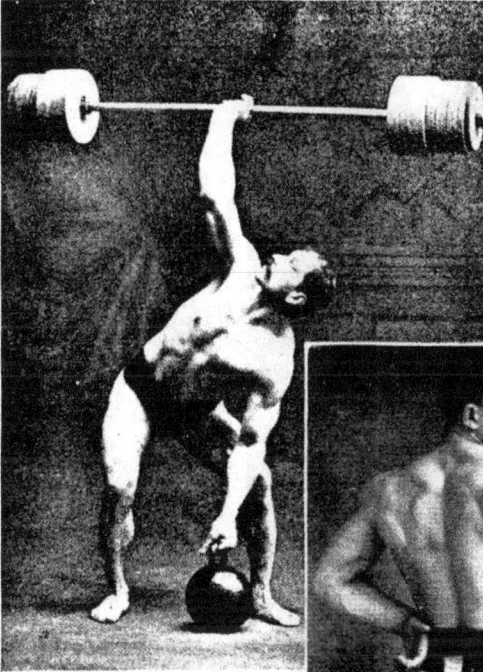

Fig. 178

Figure 178 (below)
H e r m a n   Saxon
who is neither a[
big nor as strong a[
his older brother
but has a far mor[
attractive build.

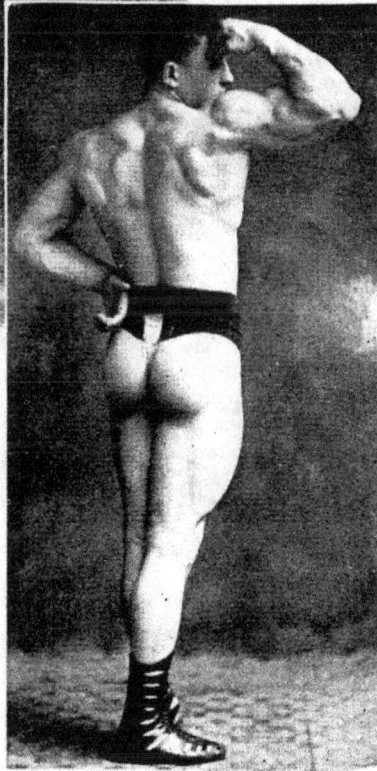

Fig. 177

Plate 92, Figure 177 (above).
Arthur Saxon making the lift
k n o w n   a s   t h e   two-hand
"Anyhow." His best record in
this lift is 448 lbs. He first
pressed aloft with his right
arm a bar-bell weighing 336
lbs.; and then leaning over, as
shown in the picture, he picked
up a 112-lb. kettle-bell in his
left hand, and after standing
erect, pushed the kettle-bell to
arm's length overhead.

269

PLATE 93

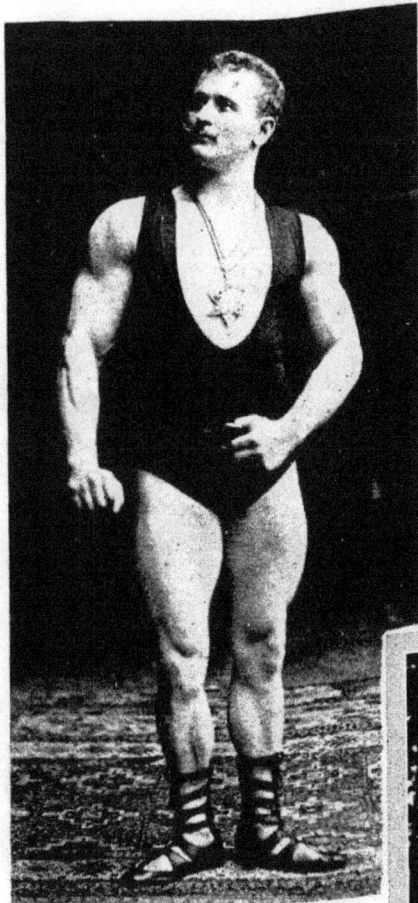

Fig. 179

Plate 93, Figure 179 (above).
A picture of Eugene Sandow
taken about 1893, which was
when he did his best lifting.
Sandow must be nearly sixty
years old at the present time,
and he is still in splendid
physical condition. Undoubtedly, he owes his present
health, strength, and vigor to
the strenuous exercise he
took as a young man

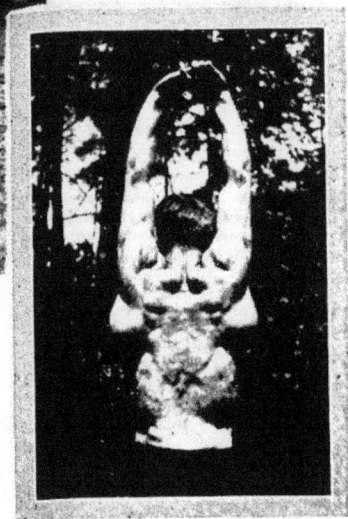

Fig. 180

Figure 180 (below). Jack Staton,
of Vancouver, in a pose which
shows his remarkable control of the
upper-back muscles

270

PLATE 94

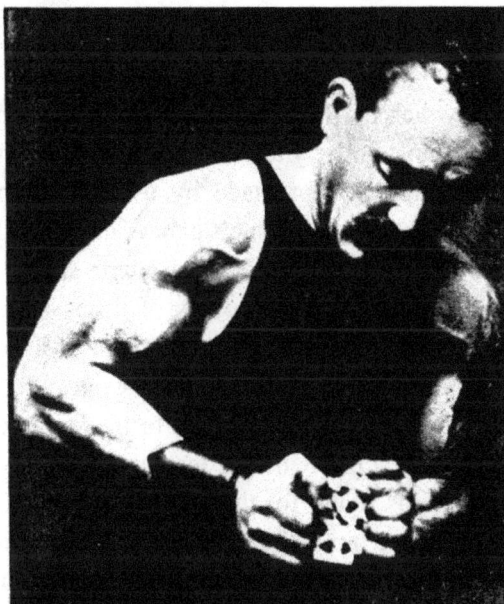

Fig. 181

Plate 94, Figure
181 (a b o v e),
Pierre Gasnier
tearing two packs
of cards

Fig. 182

Figure 182 (be-
low), G a s n i e r
doing a chain-
breaking s t u n t.
This famous ath-
lete, who recently
died of old age,
was one of the
most skillful and
scientific lifters
in the history of
the game. He was
at his best about
thirty years ago

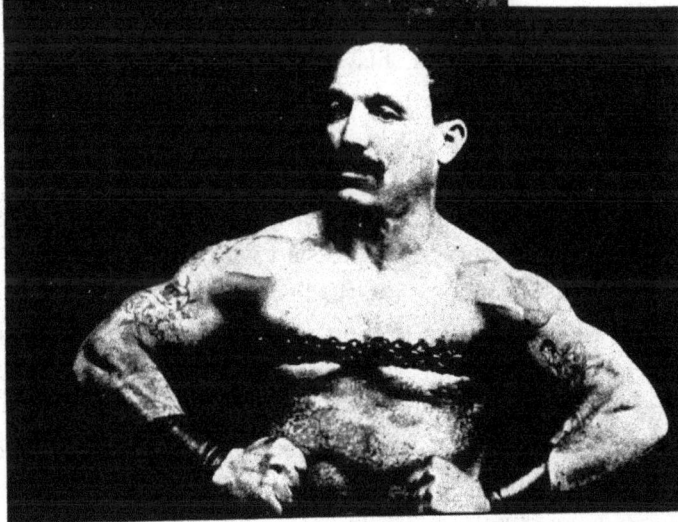

CHAPTER XXV

STATUESQUE DEVELOPMENT

The great popularity which bar-bell exercise has achieved in the last few years is due almost entirely to one feature; and that is the phenomenal physical improvement made by users of barbells. In this country, lifting is not a major sport as it is in some of the European countries. In fact, it isn't even a minor sport. You almost never see in the papers any accounts of lifting-matches, and yet there are thousands of men and boys who prefer lifting to any other kind of sport, and who prefer bar-bell exercise to any other means of body-building. This is hardly to be wondered at after you have learned that a bar-bell user increases his muscular development, and alters his figure for the better at such a rate of speed that he can almost see himself grow from one week-end to another. The devotee of light exercise is highly gratified if he increases his chest measurement by 2 inches, his arm measurement by 1 inch, his bodily weight by 5 lbs., and his strength by twenty- five percent. After a man has used a bar-bell three or four times a week over a period of six months, he is justifiably disappointed if his chest has increased less than 6 inches, his arms less than 2½ inches, and his thighs less than 3 inches. If he was very skinny to start with, he will probably have gained anywhere from 25 to 40 lbs. in good solid muscle. If he was fat when he started to train, he is not satisfied unless he has reduced his waist measurement by 8 or 10 inches. Such extraordinary improvement is not made by everyone who practices this form of exercise, but when a man fails to make those improvements, he can depend on it that the fault is with him, and not with the method.

I have become so accustomed to seeing complete physical transformation in a comparatively short space of time, that I am not only surprised, but actually grieved, when an enthusiast fails to make the gains he should have made. When such a thing happens, the investigation shows that the disappointed individual has deliberately hampered his own progress by specializing on arm and shoulder work, instead of adopting the all-round program which results in a bigger chest, broader shoulders, and a general readjustment of the lines of the figure. That, by the way, is one reason why this book is written. The fascination of lifting weights above the head is so great, that it is necessary to remind enthusiasts that by neglecting their back, loins, sides, and thighs, they are deliberately hampering their bodily growth; and actually preventing their arms from becoming as strong as they could be.

There was a time when I would get startled if a man wrote me and said that he had increased his chest measurement 6 inches in six months, but I have gotten over that. I have actually seen a slender youth increase his chest measurement from 29 to 36 inches in a little over a month's time. I have seen a tall, slender man, whose chest was no larger than his waist, so alter his proportions that at the end of a year his chest was 12 inches larger than his waist; and, at that, his waist was 2 inches larger than formerly. Mind you, he was thirty years old when he started. I have seen fat men over forty-five years old start at bar-bell work, and inside of six months so improved themselves that their bodily proportions would compare favorably with those of any of the beautifully-built athletes whose pictures illustrate this volume. I have seen puny sixteen-year-old schoolboys increase so rapidly in strength and development that inside of a year they achieved nation-wide fame for the beauty of their proportions and for their immense muscular development. I have seen a long, rangy office worker, of no particular strength, become one of the best amateur lifters in the world, and when he started he was nearly thirty. Like most of the others, he got a 44-inch chest, a 16-inch upper arm, and other measurements in proportion. It would take several books to even briefly mention the startling cases which have come under my observation.

Years ago I started to tabulate the measurements of bar-bell users, so as to get an idea of the bodily proportions which could be attained. I published my conclusions in a magazine, and subsequently they had to be published in the form of a pamphlet[1], and I understand that it has been very widely distributed, and has been accepted in many quarters as a standard.

I was familiar with a number of tables of so-called "ideal measurements" which had been compiled by artists, sculptors, physicians, and various authorities on bodily proportions. According to my ideas the measurements given in these tables were less than those possessed by many bar-bell users of my acquaintance. So I sat down and worked out my standard, and found that it was much higher than the standard given by the other writers on the subject. For example, it was claimed that a well-proportioned man of 5 feet 8 inches should have a 40-inch chest; whereas I knew lots of beautifully shaped and not overly big men of that height whose normal chests measured 43 to 44 inches. There are some who have claimed that my standard represents over-development, and that the true beauty of the figure is better represented by the ancient Greek statues. In order to discover the truth in the matter, I had a lot of these statues measured, and found that in most cases the statue came very much closer to equaling my stand- and than the more slender standards previously published. When we measured the statue of the Apollo Belvedere, we found, for example, that a man six feet tall, built on those lines, would have a chest measuring 38¼ inches, waist 31 inches, hips 36, thigh 23½ inches; neck 16

[1]This pamphlet is called, "How Much Should I Measure and How Much Should I Weigh?" and you can obtain a copy by applying to the publishers of this book.

inches, calf 11½ inches, wrist 8¼ inches, and upper arm about 15 inches. The Apollo Belvedere is supposed to represent the slender figure, but in this case the effect of slenderness was deliberately created by the sculptor when he made the trunk small, and the arms and legs large in comparison. There are lots of present-day six-footers who have chests measuring 38¼ inches, but very few of them have 15-inch upper arms, and 23½ inch thighs, and almost none of them have wrists measuring more than 8 inches.

In measuring some of the other statues of Greek athletes, we found that if the statue showed a man 5 feet 8 inches tall, the chest measurement would be 44 inches, the thigh more than 24 inches, the upper arm 16 inches, and so on. People rave about these ancient Greek athletes, and say how beautifully proportioned they were, and how smooth their muscles were; yet the measurements taken show that these apparently smoothly-built men have the measurements and the proportions of a modern "Strong Man." If you try to make yourself "built like a Greek statue," you will find that you have to make yourself very much bigger and more powerfully developed than you are at present. If a sculptor was to make an absolutely accurate statue of a tennis player or a distance-runner, that statue would look almost scrawny compared with the statues of the ancient Greeks. I commend this idea to the particular consideration of those who apparently think that the build of the tennis-player and distance-runner is the ideal build.

I find that there are many physical culturists who have the mistaken opinion that a "Strong Man" or a weight-lifter has muscles which stand out in knots and ridges even when they are relaxed. Such is not the case. Most of the lifters whom I know have muscles which are smooth and round when relaxed, but very prominent when flexed. Their muscles look equally well in either state, because their bodily proportions are so perfect. Look at Fig. 119, and you will see Anton Matysek standing at ease. Not one muscle is flexed, and consequently his body looks perfectly smooth. His proportions are so perfect that he does not have to flex his muscles in order to look impressive, but just the same the muscles are there. Look at Fig. 120, and you see him displaying his muscles. In this pose he has deliberately flexed as many muscles as possible. The two pictures were taken within ten minutes of each other. In this book there are pictures of several dozen bar-bell users, and it would be interesting to show two pictures of each man, one standing at ease, and the other one with his muscles flexed. You would want no better proof, that when the bar-bell user stands at ease his muscles are just as smooth as those of a boxer, although his bodily proportions are infinitely better. Matysek, whose pictures are shown, was much sought for as an artist's model, and has posed for many of the greatest sculptors.

It would be still more interesting to publish the pictures of the men before and after they had developed their bodies. I have many such pictures, but no room to publish them here. Unfortunately most men never think of having their pictures taken when they start to train, because they have no idea that they will be able to make any great change in their appearance. After they commence to get some development, they do have pictures taken. To give you an idea of what some of these men accomplish, I call your attention to Figs. 122 and 123, showing Mr. Woodrow before and after he used bar-bells; Figs. 124 and 125, showing Mr. Hedlund, and Figs. 126 and 127, showing Mr. Ruckstool. (The first picture of Ruckstool was taken after he had been training for five or six months, and had already made good gains. The second picture shows how he appeared a year after the first picture was taken.)

In my collection I have hundreds, and perhaps thousands, of pictures of finely developed men; a few of which are printed on the following pages. If you take the trouble to study these pictures, you will see that all these men show a certain similarity of figure, and that in some respects their development and proportions are quite different from the development and proportions of the average athlete. The same thing is noticeable about the old Greek statues. Ninety per cent of them show men of the same type; that is to say, the shoulders will be of a certain breadth in proportion to the height, the body will have a certain length in proportion to the legs; and the girth of the arms and the legs show a certain fixed proportion to the girth of the chest and hips. If you were to judge by the statues that still remain, it would be natural to assume that these Greeks represented the finest type of development to which the human race has yet attained. My own belief is that these statues represent only the very best men of their time; just as our own sculptors use only the best developed and shapely men as models. The "Greek type" of body has by no means vanished. There are plenty of athletes today who are just as well proportioned and just as beautifully developed as any Greek statue you or I have ever seen. On one occasion I showed a part of my collection to a noted sculptor, and after he had examined them thoroughly, he said, "This is the finest built lot of men I have ever seen. Apparently by your methods you can turn out men like the ancient Greek athletes. I am interested to know that such a thing is possible."

Unquestionably, the development a man can attain is dependent on the underlying bone structure; which makes it seem as though it were impossible for a small-boned man to acquire as big and powerfully developed body as is possible in the case of a man with bigger and heavier bones. The way it works out is that a man with unusually heavy bones, when properly trained, will acquire the figure and development of a Hercules; that a man of average bones will get a development of a Treseus, Perseus, or Mars; and that a small-boned man, when his figure is fully developed, will show the proportions of an Apollo or a Mercury.

277

Most men are "just average" to start with. Not more than five men out of one hundred have 6-inch wrists, and not more than two or three men out of one hundred will have 8-inch wrists. Sixty or seventy men out of one hundred will have wrists measuring somewhere between 6¼ inches and 7¼ inches. I have found that a 6¾- inch wrist is the average size for men who have sedentary occupations, while the laborers, the mechanics, or the outdoor men average a 7-inch wrist measurement.

Many of our greatest "Strong Men" have wrists measuring only 7 inches, and some of the shorter athletes have smaller wrists than that. Very small bones would seem to be a bar to pronounced muscular development, although I have seen men with very small wrists develop wonderful arms. For example, Robert Snyder, Fig. 128, whose wrist measures only 6 inches, has a 14½ inch upper arm. As he stands only 5 feet 5 inches in height, his arm looks very large. I have seen taller men, with the same size wrist, get even bigger arms than Snyder's. Thomas Inch, of London, who stands 5 feet 10 inches, who has a small hand and a 7-inch wrist, actually succeeded in developing an 18¼ inch upper arm. As a middleweight, his arm measured only 16½ inches, and his arm got to be 19 inches around when he put on 40 lbs. of weight, and moved into the heavy-weight class. There are lots of men with 7-inch wrists whose arms measure more than 16 inches in girth. Inch had to work harder to get his big arm than men like Hackenschmidt, and the Nord- quests, whose wrists measured 8 inches, and whose arms are about the same size as Inch's.

In the last part of this book you will find pictures of thirty or forty beautifully proportioned and splendidly developed athletes, and in selecting these pictures I deliberately picked men who were average-sized, and who had average-sized bones when they started to train. In looking over these pictures, you will notice a marked similarity in the shape of the muscles. The 16-inch arms of one of these athletes will look almost exactly like the 16-inch arms of another athlete. In fact, the resemblance in development is so marked, that if you concealed the faces, it would be hard to tell some of the men apart. That is because they are the uniform product of a uniform system of training. The reason their bodies look alike is because their bodies are perfectly developed; and perfectly developed muscles almost assume a certain size, shape, and outline. Therefore, if you have average-sized bones, and take up the same system of training which these men used, you will acquire just the type of physique represented in these pictures. Some of these men, especially the professionals, like Saxon, and Hackenschmidt, were strong and above the average in build to start with; but the rest of the amateurs were no better when they started than you are now; or than nine out of ten men of your acquaintance. That is why I am so strongly impressed with the value of bar-bell exercise as a means of body-building.

You will have to admit that the men, whose pictures appear on these pages, are vastly superior in sheer bodily beauty to men developed by any other form of exercise or athletics. No group of oarsmen, football players, runners, wrestlers, or gymnasts could show proportions or development equal to that possessed by these bar-bell users. The only sport which produces a type of physique anything like this is ground-tumbling. A combination of tumbling and hand-balancing will yield a fine development. It is noteworthy that almost all bar-bell users do a certain amount of hand-balancing and tumbling. It seems that after a man has used bar-bells for a while he acquires such strength and agility that he can take up the other two sports, and by reason of his physical advantages, quickly become a star tumbler, or a star hand-balancer. On the other hand, men who have practiced nothing except tumbling and hand-balancing frequently take up bar-bell work in order to acquire the extra bodily strength which will make them better performers in their own line of work.

But go back to the pictures. In each one of these men you will see that he has a certain shoulder-breadth in proportion to his height; that his chest is not only wide from side to side, but deep from front to back. In the back-view pictures you will see a great display of muscles from one shoulder to another and, more important still, two great cables of muscle along either side of the spine in the lower part of the back. In the front-view pictures you will see that the abdominal muscles, which are never visible in the average man, are here clearly outlined. In some of these pictures you will be able to see the muscles at the sides of the waist. The legs are differently shaped from those of the average man. There is far more muscle on the outside of the thigh, while on the back of the thigh there is a swelling outward curve, which you will find only in strong-backed men like these. If the picture is taken from the side, you will see that the front of the thigh shows a pronounced curve starting right above the knee, and ending at the hip.

You can find pictures of gymnasts with equally big arms; you may find some pictures of outdoor athletes and tumblers who have legs almost as good, but you positively will not find any other class of athlete who can equal the bar-bell user in symmetrical development from head to heel. The development of the lower part of the trunk (that is, the waist, the loins, the hips), and the development of the thighs, which bar-bell users and weight-lifters possess, cannot be found in any other type of athlete; because this kind of development is not produced by any other form of physical activity. Nevertheless, it is just the kind of development and just the kind of outlines you see in the old Greek statues.

There are some authorities on the subject of muscular development who claim that a weight-lifter's muscles are "short," and those people express their preference for what we call "long, elastic muscles." (This is a question which I have

280

discussed a number of times in various magazine articles.) The length of a muscle is governed by the length of the nearby bones. For instance, the biceps muscle is fastened at its lower end to the bone of the forearm, and one of its upper ends to the bone of the upper arm, and the other end to the bone which forms the shoulder girdle. Therefore, if a man has attained his full growth, which means that the upper arm bone has stopped growing, it is impossible to either shorten or lengthen the biceps muscle. Naturally, muscle becomes shorter and thicker as it contracts, which explains why your biceps rise in a swelling curve when you bend the arm. Similarly, a muscle lengthens as it relaxes or is extended; but you cannot make your muscle longer no matter what you do, unless you make the bone of the upper arm longer. The bigger a muscle is the shorter is looks. A six-footer, with narrow shoulders and thin arms, appears to have very long arms, but if, by exercise, he increases the width of his shoulders by 3 or 4 inches, and adds as many inches to the girth of his arm then his arm will appear to be much shorter than it was before because it is thicker. Any man with undeveloped arms appears to have long arm muscles, and it is perfectly true that a man with a perfect development appears to have short arm muscles. In the undeveloped man the deltoid muscle on the point of the shoulder is so small in size that it fails to make itself apparent. In a well- developed man the deltoid muscles are thick and quite prominent. Look at the pictures of Charles Durner, Fig. 121. In his left arm you can see the deltoid muscle coming down to a point more than one-third down the upper arm. This muscle overlays part of the biceps and the triceps muscles of the upper arm. Therefore, Durner's arm muscles look short because their upper ends are concealed by the fully developed deltoid. Also, his forearms are powerfully developed, and in the left arm the forearm muscle runs up across the bottom of the biceps, and that helps to make the upper arm look shorter. His right arm is so powerfully developed that it looks short in proportion to its length, but if you will bear the foregoing statements in mind, you can see how the right deltoid overlaps the upper end of the biceps, and how the muscle o n the inside of the right forearm cuts the line of the biceps at its lower end. If Durner's arms were thin, his muscles would appear to be long, but really they are still just as long as before he got his development, and they are far more elastic than they were when he started to train.

It will be interesting for you to go over all these pictures and study the effect of the deltoid on the appearance of the arm. You will not be able to find a single weak-looking deltoid muscle, and in many cases you will find that the deltoid is so splendidly developed that you can follow its outlines almost as clearly as though the skin had been removed. In some of the back-view pictures, where the hands are raised above the head, the deltoid muscles are very prominent, as in the picture of Adolph Nordquest. Fig. 6. The muscles are seen almost equally clear when the athlete is holding a heavy weight in his hands. Look at the deltoids of Steinborn, Fig. 130, and Donald, Fig. 15. While we are on the subject of shoulders, I suggest that you study the appearance of the trapezius muscles, which lie on the upper back at the base of the neck, and which form the line at the top of the shoulders. Any real strong man has to have the trapezius muscles developed to a high extent, and that is why weight lifters have sloping shoulders. If you see a man whose shoulders apparently go out in straight lines from the base of the neck, that man is weak. In a picture of Paschall, Fig. 132, the shoulders appear to go out in just that way, but that is because Paschall, after folding his arms, slightly shrugged his shoulders and spread them apart. Just the same, you can see the line of the trapezius muscle running from the right side of his neck toward the right deltoid. If Paschall allowed his arms to hang at his sides, his shoulders would be just as sloping as those of Sigmund Klein (in Fig. 133), or of Steinborn (in Fig. 130).

In all the pictures you will see how the body tapers from the line of the armpits to the waist. Without looking up their measurements, I would say offhand that every one of these men has a normal chest measurement 10 inches larger than his waist measurement. In some of the pictures the difference appears even greater. That is because the athlete has spread his shoulders by the method described in the chapter "Muscle Control." In the picture of Matysek, Fig. 134, the tapering effect is caused partly by the twist of the body. Any well-developed man can approximate this effect by standing as Matysek does. (The secret of the pose is to twist the body until the shoulders are practically at right angles with the hips. If you allow your hips to twist, the tapering effect is lost.) This picture is very interesting, because it shows the enormous size of the latissimus muscle on the right side of Matysek's back. The name "latissimus dorsi" means the broad-of-the-back, and in this picture it certainly justifies its name. Unless those muscles are fully developed, the back will not taper, no matter how broad your shoulders are. This can be proved by observing any tall man with broad shoulders. If he is undeveloped, the breadth of his shoulders comes entirely from the size of his bony framework, and his sides will be straight up and down. If, however, he has a proper back development, his back will be considerably wider at the line of his arm-pits than at the line of his waist.

In studying the pictures of any well-developed man, you should always try to get an idea of the depth of his chest, and in order to do that you have to see both the front and the back lines of the body. It is possible for almost any fairly developed man to make himself look as though he had a deep chest when a picture is being taken. This is done by hollowing the back, and pushing the chest out, and then holding the arms close to the side so that the hollow back is concealed. A man with a really deep chest doesn't have to resort to that trick.

The reason these men have such good forearms is because when handling bar-bells the forearm muscles are employed in almost every exercise. About the only exception is when you lay the bar-bell across the shoulders and "squat" to develop the legs. In all the arm exercises, all the shoulder exercises, the tack exercises, and in some of the leg exercises the bell is held in the hands and. consequently, the muscles of the forearms and the hands have to contract vigorously. In all the exercise, when the arm is bent (as when developing the biceps), the forearm muscles are subjected to considerable work in helping to bend the arm. (This was discussed in Chapter XIII.)

The size of your upper arm is more or less influenced by the size of your forearm, and both parts of the arm should be developed at the same time. You can get a fair development of the forearms by clinching the fingers; that is, doing gripping exercises, and by twisting the wrist, but those exercises don't produce nearly as big muscles, or nearly as strong muscles, as when you have to grip a heavy object in the hands and then bend the arms at the elbows. Furthermore, merely gripping with the fingers will not produce as strong a grip as lifting heavy objects with the hands. When you do the "Jefferson" lift, Fig. 18, you will develop a far stronger grip than you can get by opening and closing the fingers against no resistance. When you do the two variations of the two-arm "curl" for developing the biceps you will develop the upper part of your forearms in a way that you never will by simply twisting the wrists. The arm should be developed as a unit, and not as separate parts. The reason the arms of these men look so well-knit is because many of their exercises have required them to use their muscles in the hand, arm, and shoulder at the same time.

The general rule is that the flexed biceps should be twenty per cent larger than the forearm, and most of these men show that proportion. The only great exception is Anton Matysek, who

284

could never get his forearms above 12½ inches, although his upper arms measured 16½ inches. Yet Matysek's forearms and wrists were extraordinarily strong, as was proven when he beat Joe Nordquest in a back-hand "curl" with a thick handled bar-bell. Usually, when a man has small forearms, the calves of his legs are likewise small. This was not so in Matysek's case, because his calves measured 16 inches. The peculiar thing was that they were very deep from front to back, and only moderately wide.

No one can handle bar-bells without developing wonderful deltoid muscles. As you were previously told, the deltoid lifts the arm. The reason a bar-bell user's deltoids are so big and shapely, is because he develops his triceps by pushing the bar-bell overhead; whereas the gymnast develops his triceps by pushing the hands downward, as when "dipping" on the parallel bars, and the ordinary physical culturist develops his triceps by pushing the hands forward, as when doing the "floor dip." (This dipping develops the muscles on the front of the chest far more than it does the deltoids on the points of the shoulders.)

Without fine deltoids you will never look impressive, either when you have your pictures taken or when you appear on the floor of the "gym" or on the bathing beach. Properly developed deltoid muscles in some way give a peculiar appearance of manliness by adding to the squareness of the shoulders, and by enhancing the arm development. With poor deltoids you will never look strong, even if your arms are big and your chest muscles big; but fine deltoids are the finishing touch which gives the effect of great strength and athletic ability.

The hips and thighs are just as worthy of study as are the arms and shoulders, and, in fact, are a better indication of bodily strength. Just as the upper-arm muscles should merge into the muscles of the shoulder, so should the muscles of the thighs merge into the hips. In a properly developed leg the thigh should taper from the crotch to the knee. Many gymnasts and physical culturists show some development of the lower part of the thigh, but little development near the hips. In outdoor men just the reverse is the case. There are some men who show no muscle at all on the back of the thigh; others who have so little muscle on the inside of the thighs that when they stand with their knees touching, the thighs fail to touch by an inch; still others have no development on the outside of the thigh.

Notice that in a good many of these pictures it is hard to tell where the thighs stop and the hips begin. In a picture of Owen Carr, Fig. 136, the front line of his right thigh seems to run right to his waist. You see such development only in a man who has an equally fine development of the muscles on the front of the abdomen; therefore you never see a fat man with a leg like Carr's. In pictures like those of Nordquest, Matysek and some of the others you see a very pronounced curve on the outside of the thigh. This is partly due to the fact that they turned their toes slightly outward when having their pictures taken, but even when they stand with the toes pointed straight forward, their thighs show almost as great a development in the vastus externus; that is, the outer muscle of the thigh. In every such case you will find above the thighs powerfully developed muscles at the sides of the waist. Most of the men who show this pronounced development got it from practicing the side exercise, Fig. 33, and later on the one-arm "bent press."

A man with a big biceps muscle on the back of the thighs always has big and powerful muscles on the small of the back.

In the three foregoing paragraphs you will find the real explanation of the extraordinary bodily strength of these men. Great thigh strength and great strength in the waist always go together. Of all of these men, hardly one of them shows a thigh

286

measurement of less than 23 inches, and some of them have thighs measuring 26 inches around. None of them has a waist less than 30 inches or more than 34 inches. It is that uniformity of measurements in so many different men which enables me to say so confidently that any man of average size and weight, with average-sized bones, can get the kind of development which these pictures show.

CHAPTER XXVI

EFFECTS OF EXERCISE

A man who possesses super-strength also commands a good deal of admiration. The general public worships physical strength. The announcement of a celebrated "Strong Man" to appear at a vaudeville theater insures that there will be "standing room only" during the term of his engagement. Most people rate great physical strength higher than speed or suppleness; although there are a certain number of folk who affect to sneer at what they call the "truck horse" type of development. The pictures on these pages should convince anyone that a man can become wonderfully strong without becoming overly heavy or clumsy in appearance.

It is true that some of the old-time "Strong Men" could justly have been called "truck horses." Louis Cyr, Horace Barre, and one or two of their contemporaries were men who had enormous frames, and those bodies were of the bulky type. Swaboda, of Vienna, is about the only modern "Strong Man" who comes in that class.

Now, I admire strength as much as anyone does, but I do not consider strength to be so important that one should sacrifice speed, agility, or suppleness in becoming strong. Happily, modern training methods seem to produce a combination of all the most desirable physical gifts. In support to this statement, I refer to the accompanying pictures. Outside of the three old-timers referred to above, you will not find a man here who is clumsy in appearance, or who looks as though he would be slow in his movements. Activity depends almost as much on bodily proportions as it does on the nervous organization. It has been claimed that a man of placid, sluggish temperament is never quick in movement. That may or may not be true, although it does seem to be a fact that many intensely nervous and highly strung individuals are very quick both in their mental processes and their bodily movement. There are athletic coaches who will tell you that all weight- lifters are slow, and that the practice of weight lifting is bound to make one slow. My answer to this is that those particular gentlemen have never seen any first-class modern lifters. As a rule, the highly developed weight-lifter does not know the meaning of nerves. Such men are of an extremely finely balanced temperament, and a quiet disposition. If you see such a man in his street clothes, and watch him as he moves about, you might get the impression that he was very deliberate in everything he did, and that, in turn, might make you think that he was slow. So far as I can see, all first-class lifters move just that way; but theirs is a calculated deliberation. They are experts in what you might call "physical economy," and rarely make one unnecessary motion. Their constant training with bar-bells has given them an uncanny sense of timing, such as is possessed among other athletes only by high-grade boxers or jugglers. I have never seen a man more quietly deliberate than Arthur Saxon; in everything he did, whether off or on the stage, he was absolutely unhurried. He never made a false motion, but he never failed to accomplish any lift which required speed. Saxon was a big-boned man, but never grew heavy. He seemed to keep his average weight of 210 lbs. no matter how much or how little he ate and drank.

His younger brother, Herman, at right in Fig. 139, though somewhat lighter in build, was no quicker than Arthur. Herman, who weighed about 168 lbs., was one of the most perfectly built men I have ever seen. I have sometimes thought that, although he was noticeably less strong than Arthur, he was much more admired as an athlete.

If you should take up bar-bell exercise with the avowed intention of becoming super-strong, you need not waste any time worrying about the danger of getting a build like Cyr's. He was always big, and always fleshy. I suppose that few of you would object to getting a build like that of Herman Saxon, of Sandow, of Adolph Nordquest, of Steinborn, of Carr, or Matysek. All those just named are big men; but they are big without being bulky; powerfully developed without being slow or clumsy, and withal, noticeably graceful in build. The back-view picture of Adolph Nordquest, Fig. 141, does not look like the portrait of a slow or clumsy man, and the appearance of lightness is due to his proportions. The man has a tremendous frame, and if he had a big waist (like Cyr's) he would look slow and clumsy, but the picture shows that his waist is obviously considerably smaller than his hips, and very much smaller than his chest. Few men are as strong as he. He can made a one-arm "press" with a 250-lb. bar-bell, and he can lift as much weight off the ground as any professional I have ever seen. He is one of the best in the world at the standing broad jump, and at the time this picture was taken could run 100 yards in ten seconds without training. He does not look to be extraordinarily big, because he is so perfectly proportioned, and yet his chest measures about 46 inches, his upper arm over 17 inches, and his thigh about 26 inches; but not one part of him seems to be overdeveloped. I defy you to look at that picture and pick out a weak spot on his anatomy. His build is so similar to Sandow's that for several years he worked under the name of "Young Sandow," and the resemblance between the two men was so startling that many people thought that Nordquest was Sandow's younger brother.

If your bones are above the average in size; that is, if you have a 7½-inch wrist, and 9½-inch ankle, bar-bell work will give you a build something like Nordquest's, but there is no danger of giving you a build like Cyr's. I would not advise anyone to exercise with weights if I thought for one moment that such training was likely to produce a body which was bulky without being shapely, or which would create strength at the expense of speed and suppleness. It is true that Cyr's lifting records were better than Nordquest's, but not very much better. I, for one, would much prefer to have the shape and the combined strength and speed of an Adolph Nordquest to the mere bulk and power of a Cyr.

Steinborn is another very big man. He is probably an inch shorter than Adolph Nordquest, and five pounds heavier. His measurements are just as big, but his muscular development is not as pronounced. If anything, he is slightly quicker in his movements than even Nordquest; which may be due to the fact that Nordquest, in his training, specialized on what we call "slow presses" and "dead-weight lifting," whereas Steinborn has practiced almost exclusively at the "quick lifts." Although nearly 100 lbs. lighter than Cyr, Steinborn is capable of breaking most of Cyr's records. The best Cyr ever put up with one arm was 273 lbs., and he used a "slow press"; furthermore, the bell he put up was not as heavy as he was himself. I am positive that Steinborn could put up close to 300 lbs. in a one-arm "jerk," and that is about ten per cent more than any other athlete in history has put up by the same method. Steinborn is a refutation of the theory that the use of bar-bells and continued lifting produces short knotted muscles, and makes one slow. If you will look at Fig. 142, you get the impression of a man of immense power, but you will not see any knotted muscles. Steinborn's development is as smooth as that of a boxer. The man has a tremendous arm, although it does not look very big in this pose, on account of the great spread of the man's shoulders.

You might think that if a man is very heavy to start with, that the effect of the training would be to make him still heavier, or that if he started with a 48-inch chest and a 46-inch waist, his chest might increase to 52 inches and his waist get even bigger than it was before. Just the opposite happens. When a stout man starts to train, the first visible effect is that he becomes smaller instead of bigger. Any tailor will tell you that a 44-inch chest is extraordinarily big for a small-waisted man, but that some of his stout customers—the fellows with the big waists—have chests measuring nearly 50 inches. When your waist gets abnormally large, all the near-by parts are affected; the hips become bulky, the upper part of the thighs get so big that they "interfere"; the arms get fat close to where they join the shoulders, and big folds of flesh make their appearance on the upper part of the chest. If a man started with a 48-inch chest and a 46-inch waist, it is probable that his chest measurement would decrease to about 43 inches, while his waist measurement was decreasing to 36 inches. As soon as he commenced to give vigorous work to the muscles of the upper body, the extra fat in those parts would disappear; and in the stout man, such as the one described, that extra fat is responsible for several inches of his chest measurement. After he had gotten rid of this fat, his chest would go back to 46 or maybe to 48 inches, as he increased the size of the rib-box, and the development, and consequent thickness, of the upper-body muscles. In some cases the chest does not grow smaller as the waist decreases. The muscles develop so rapidly that they fill up the space left by the disappearing fatty tissue.

Naturally, there are very few stout men who train for muscular development. With most of them the only idea is to become smaller. In the average fat man, a reduction of 10 inches in waist measurement is accompanied with a decrease in the size of the chest, the upper arms, and the upper part of the thighs. Men like Cyr and Barry were more or less abnormal, whereas men like Adolph Nordquest and Steinborn have an absolute normal development ; that is, the shape and size of their muscles is exactly what it should be in proportion to the underlying bones. I have superintended the training of many fat men, and I never saw one of them grow to be anything like Cyr in shape; although I have seen many first reduce themselves, and then develop a figure of the Nordquest-Steinborn type.

But that is all special work. Seven out of ten men have average sized bones, are of average height, and of average measurements; therefore, if ten men read this chapter, seven of them are concerned with what can be done for the average man. Every week I personally inspect measurement charts of at least one hundred men, and it is safe to say that in the last ten years I have studied over fifty thousand sets of charts. In doing this kind of work you absorb a great deal of information. I have gotten so that if you tell me a man's height and weight, I can come very close to telling you the measurements of his chest, arms, legs, and so on. If you tell me a man's measurements, and his height, I can tell you just about how much he weighs.

I do not know whether these figures would apply in accurate proportion to the male population, but I do know that the average measurements of thousands of physically cultured who start training with bar-bells,—are a 36-inch chest, 12½-inch upper arm, 10½ -inch forearm, 6½ -inch wrist, 20-inch thigh, and so on. If you have such measurements you can say, "Well, I am as big as the average," and if you are satisfied with average development, that is as far as you go. I have always contended that the average man has much less development, and very much less strength than he should have, and evidently there is a certain proportion of the public that agrees with me. Otherwise, why should so many of these average men be so anxious to start at a training program to make themselves bigger, better developed, and stronger?

It is a mistake to confuse the words "average" and "normal." The "average development" is not necessarily the "normal development." My opinion is that instead of the average development being the normal development, and the development of the weight lifter being abnormal, the exact opposite is the case. The weight lifter's development is absolutely normal, and what every man should have, and can have; the average development is subnormal.

The brain power of a great scientist or a great mathematician is not abnormal in any way, although it is far greater than the brain power of a man whose education was confined to what he got in the elementary schools. The scientist, by reason of his work, is continually cultivating his brain power, because he is continually using his brain. If he goes on a vacation, or stops his work or study, he may forget some special bits of information, but he does not lose any of his reasoning power. If a man deliberately takes up a good training system to develop his muscles, and if he gets results (such as were gotten by the men whose pictures you see here), he does not become abnormal, but simply shows what is possible in the way of cultivated bodily improvements. If he has trained along the right lines, he retains his increased health, strength, and development long after he stops training.

It is generally accepted that Eugen Sandow, as a young man, was as beautifully proportioned and as finely developed as any man of recent times. When he first went to England, he was frequently interviewed by newspaper men. One reporter asked him how he got his development. In reply he said, "When I was a young man, I was a mere stripling, and thought to strengthen my frame by a little light exercise, like the working of a wooden wand, or a light iron bar. This loosened all my muscles and made them pliant, but no great amount of development came from the exercises. This set me thinking, and I gradually found out what exercises were the best to develop certain kinds of muscles. Using my knowledge with the weights I had at my command, I began to gradually increase my weights, and soon found out that I could easily put up a 100-lb. dumbbell. This interview was reprinted in a book which Sandow wrote in 1894. In the same book he said, "The dumbbell and the bar-bell have been my chief means of physical training." When he made those statements he was at the height of his power and development, and it should be specially noted that this was several years before the appearance of the so- called "grip dumbbell," which is so widely associated with his name. In another interview reprinted in his first book, he was asked whether he observed severe rules regarding diet. In reply he said, "I just eat and drink what I want, when I want, and in what quantities I want"

World-famous "Strong Men," like Saxon and Steinborn, ascribe all their strength to the use of bar-bells, and state in the most positive terms that they consider any other kind of exercises to be a mere waste of time. Their testimonials could be supported by equally enthusiastic testimonials from every man whose picture appears in this book. No one of them was anything remarkable to start with. Most of them were of the average size I have already described;—that is, they had 36-inch chests, 12½-inch upper arms, and so on. Some few of them were a little above the average. The Nordquests, Steinborn, Massimo, and one or two others would come in that class; but men like Matysek, Carr, Tauscher, Tampke, Donald, Karasick, and all the others were no stronger and no bigger when they started than nine out of ten of the young men you will find on the floor of the Y. M. C. A. gymnasium. They all did the same kind of work, and they all got the same kind of results.

It is because I have seen so many average men improve themselves to the point where they had 44-inch chests, 16-inch upper arms, 24-inch thighs, a bodily weight of 175 lbs., and three times their former strength, that I have come to believe that such results are possible for practically every normal man of average size and average shape. If only one or two of them had increased their chest measurement from 36 to 44 inches, such a gain would have to be considered as exceptional; and possible only to certain favored individuals. The fact that so many dozens of them have made those gains seems to prove that the acquired size and strength is the normal result, and not the exceptional result. It is impossible to find any other training method which produces such uniform results, in such widely different cases, as does the scientific use of bar-bells.

I have corresponded with thousands of men and boys who are interested in bodily development, and I find that, as a rule, men are much more interested in getting perfect proportions and superb muscular development than in getting great strength. It seems to me that every man has a feeling that if he could only find the right method he could become perfectly developed, no matter how poor he might be to start with. The reason we all admire the ancient Greek statues is because we instinctively feel that here is the kind of body we should have; and which we might have if we only knew how to get it. I, myself, cannot draw a picture of a perfectly built man, but the minute I see a photograph I can tell you whether the subject is, or is not, perfectly built; and, in the second case, what he would have to do to get perfect proportions. Most of you possess the same ability. If you examine the picture of an athlete you will probably say, "I do not like that fellow's build. He is top heavy. His arms and shoulders are grand, but his legs are too thin." On the other hand, you may say, "If that man's arms and chest were only anywhere nearly as fine as his legs he would have a wonderful build." If some one handed you a pencil, and asked you to make a drawing of what you considered to be a perfect build, it is possible that you could not make an accurate sketch, any more than I can; but just the same you know what you like in the way of bodily development.

The easiest way to satisfy yourself is to test your reaction when you do examine a photograph. If you at once exclaim, "My, what a man!" or "My, how splendidly that chap is built!", then you can rest assured that the man is perfectly proportioned from head to foot. But if, when you first see the picture, you say, "What wonderful arms!" or "What wonderful legs!", it is the best possible sign that the subject of the picture is not perfectly proportioned, because you first noticed one part of his body to the exclusion of the other parts. In an absolutely perfectly proportioned body, no part is unduly prominent. If you examine parts in detail you will find that the arms are wonderful, that the legs are wonderful, the chest wonderful, and so on, but it is not until every part is equally wonderful that the build becomes so perfect that when seeing the picture you say, "What a wonderful body that man has!"

Now, that is the whole secret of the effect produced by the Greek statue. Every part of the statue is perfect in itself, but never unduly prominent. Some of the pictures in this book will stand comparison with any photographs of the old Greek statues. There are men whose pictures appear in this collection whose bodies seem to me to be without a flaw. At first inspection some of them may not seem to you to be quite as beautiful as the ancient works of art, and that is because the heads are slightly larger in proportion to the bodies. The old Greek sculptors had a trick of making their statues more impressive by making the heads slightly smaller than they actually were.

To go back to the possibilities of the average man I ask you to give a careful study to the various pictures of Anton Matysek,

Owen Carr, Alexander Karasick, E. W. Goodman, Melvin Tampke, and Robert Dallas. All of these men have the so-called "statuesque figure." All of them have bones of average size. None of them was any bigger or better developed than the average man when he started to train. The present beauty of their figures is partly due to the readjustment of the bones which form the shoulder girdle and the rib-box, and the perfect development of each and every muscle in the body. Some of these pictures are especial favorites of mine. The picture of Matysek, which appears on the frontispiece, won prizes at several photographic exhibitions by reason of the beauty of the pose and the harmonious development of the athlete himself. The picture of Owen Carr, Fig. 136, is another one of which I am particularly fond. Carr has made no effort to flex his muscles, but he makes a great impression on account of the firm way in which he is standing, plus the beautiful proportions of his figure. I like Fig. 136 very much better than the accompanying picture, Fig. 144, in which Carr has all of his muscles flexed.

Such athletes as Sigmund Klein, Ignatius Neubauer, Robert Snyder, and Ali Kotier, Fig. 145, are men slightly below the average height, although you would never suspect that fact from looking at their photographs. They appear to be just as perfectly proportioned as are the taller men, like Carr and Tampke. Of course, their measurements are not quite as large, although the pictures prove that they are perfectly developed for their height.

I close this chapter with sincere regret. I would like to go ahead and analyze all these muscle-poses. I would like to tell you about each man; how long it took him to get his development, how much he can lift, how much he measures, and so on. Each one of these men is worthy of a chapter to himself. There are pictures here of men whom I have not even had a chance to mention, although they are well worthy of special mention. I have hundreds of other pictures, many of which are as good as those

297

which are published here. Every book has a limit in size, and I have reached the limit of this one. If it has interested you, and if you wish more knowledge on the subject, I suggest that you apply to the publishers of this book; who will gladly supply you with pamphlets and booklets containing various magazine articles and special essays which I have written on the subject of bodily development and muscular strength.

CPSIA information can be obtained
at www.ICGtesting.com
Printed in the USA
LVHW042000111019
633944LV00034B/612/P

9 781475 153224